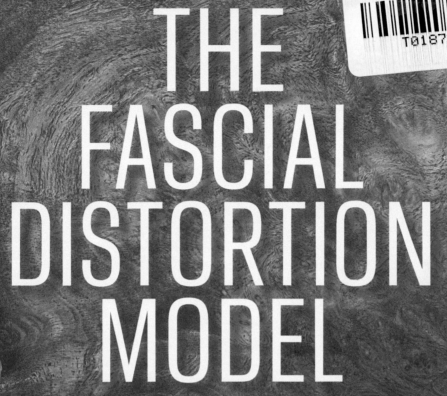

THE
FASCIAL
DISTORTION
MODEL

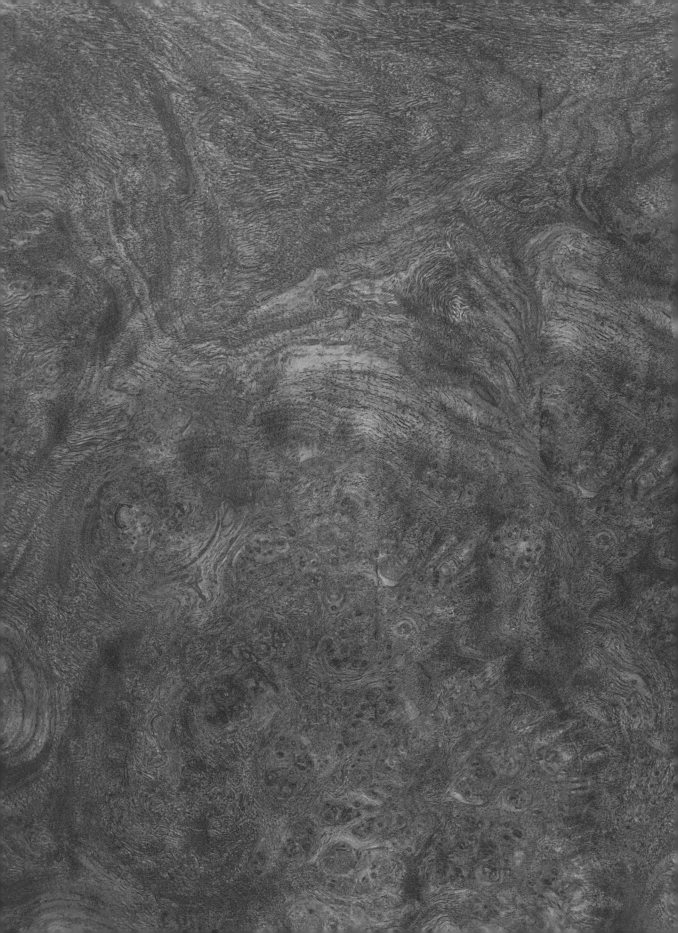

THE FASCIAL DISTORTION MODEL

Philosophy, principles, and clinical applications

Todd Capistrant ◆ Georg Harrer

Assistant Editor Thomas Pentzer

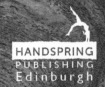

HANDSPRING
PUBLISHING
Edinburgh

HANDSPRING PUBLISHING LIMITED
The Old Manse, Fountainhall,
Pencaitland, East Lothian
EH34 5EY, Scotland
Tel: +44 1875 341 859
Website: www.handspringpublishing.com

First published 2021 in the United Kingdom by Handspring Publishing
© Handspring Publishing 2021

List of borrowed illustrations
Figures 5.1, 5.2, 5.26, 5.27, 5.34, 5.35, 5.36 © Kristen Janssen, used with kind permission.
Figure 5.10 © Nevit Dilmen, CC BY-SA 3.0, https://commons.wikimedia.org/w/index.php?curid=17361673
Figure 5.11 © Nevit Dilmen, CC BY-SA 3.0, https://commons.wikimedia.org/w/index.php?curid=17746494
Figures 5.55 and 5.66 Based on original drawings by Brianna Regan Davis, used with kind permission
Figure 15.1 © 1992 et 2013, Institut de recherche de l'Hôpital d'Ottawa 725, av. Parkdale Ottawa ON K1Y 4A9 Canada. http://www.ohri.ca/emerg/cdr/docs/cdr_ankle_poster.pdf.

ISBN 978-1-912085-56-9
ISBN (Kindle eBook) 978-1-912085-57-6

British Library Cataloguing in Publication Data
A catalogue record for this book is available from the British Library
Library of Congress Cataloging in Publication Data
A catalog record for this book is available from the Library of Congress

Notice
Neither the Publisher nor the Authors assume any responsibility for any loss or injury and/or damage to persons or property arising out of or relating to any use of the material contained in this book. It is the responsibility of the treating practitioner, relying on independent expertise and knowledge of the patient, to determine the best treatment and method of application for the patient.
All reasonable efforts have been made to obtain copyright clearance for illustrations in the book for which the authors or publishers do not own the rights. If you believe that one of your illustrations has been used without such clearance please contact the publishers and we will ensure that appropriate credit is given in the next reprint.

Commissioning Editor Mary Law
Copy Editor Fiona Conn
Project Manager Fiona Conn
Designer Bruce Hogarth
Indexer Aptara, India
Typesetter DSM, India
Printer Finidr, Czech Republic

The
Publisher's
policy is to use
paper manufactured
from sustainable forests

CONTENTS

ABOUT THE AUTHORS

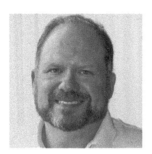

Todd Capistrant DO MHA CS is a graduate of Des Moines University, where he earned both his DO and MHA degrees. He has been active in promoting the use of the FDM since 2006 when he was first treated using the model. He has served many roles on the board of the American Fascial Distortion Model Association (AFDMA) and has served a two-term period as the organization's President. In 2010, Dr Capistrant became an instructor teaching the FDM and since then has conducted courses throughout the United States and internationally. He is a member of the Fascial Distortion Model Global Organization (FDMGO) and was one of the original signatories of the charter documents that created that organization. Dr Capistrant authored an introductory book called *Why Does it Hurt?* that introduces the FDM to anyone interested in learning the basics about this modality.

Dr Capistrant currently practices full-time Osteopathic Manipulative Medicine in Fairbanks, Alaska with Foundation Health Partners Tanana Valley Clinic. He was the founding member of a vibrant OMM department that has grown to six members and now includes a hospital practice. He credits the success of this department to the universal implementation of the FDM by all the practitioners in the group.

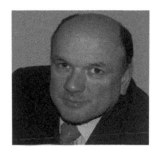

Georg Harrer MD holds a doctorate from the Medical Faculty of the University of Vienna. He is a specialist in anesthetics and intensive care, and a general practitioner. In addition to his medical studies he completed a postgraduate training in osteopathy at the Vienna School of Osteopathy (WSO). In 1997 he met Stephen P. Typaldos when the latter was invited by the WSO to hold one of his first worldwide Fascial Distortion Model (FDM) courses. The concept of FDM immediately fascinated Dr Harrer, and the following year he visited Dr Typaldos at his clinic in Maine, USA. The two men became personal friends and shared many detailed discussions on the FDM and patient care. Dr Harrer assisted at numerous FDM courses in Europe and helped with the translation of the third edition of Typaldos' FDM book into German. In 2001 Dr Typaldos authorized him to teach the FDM.

Over the years Georg Harrer has given hundreds of FDM seminars, mainly in Europe, but also in Africa and the USA. He has also contributed on the subject of FDM to several textbooks in the field of osteopathy and fascia.

In 2006 he founded the European FDM Association (EFDMA) and became its first president. In 2011 he was President of the 5th FDM World Congress in Vienna. He is a board member of FDMGO, the Global FDM Association. In addition to his international teaching activities, Dr Harrer runs a medical practice specializing in the FDM in Vienna, Austria.

PREFACE

In September of 2017, Fascial Distortion Model (FDM) practitioners from all over the world gathered in Cologne, Germany for the 7th FDM World Congress. Following days of talks delivered by skilled practitioners, we (Georg Harrer and Todd Capistrant) decided to collaborate on a new FDM textbook. Engaging in several discussions regarding the purpose of a new text, we agreed that while Dr Typaldos' textbook is the foundation of the Fascial Distortion Model, the fact that his original textbooks are not widely available presents a barrier to learning and to faithful transmission of the model to new practitioners.

Dr Typaldos created four editions of his FDM textbook before he passed away, and as his understanding of the model grew and his ideas were refined, the content of his textbooks changed. One cannot help but wonder how many editions of his book there would be today, and what the model would look like, if he had been able to continue his work.

As the model has been transmitted, we see subtle changes with each new instructor's interpretation of Dr Typaldos' original work. While we suffered a great loss with his passing, Dr Typaldos left us with two people whom he felt were qualified to teach the model as he thought it should be taught: Dr Georg Harrer and Keisuke Tanaka. Through diligence and hard work, the model continues to spread, and today there are FDM practitioners on every continent, save Antarctica (and we're working on that!) We consider preserving the key tenets of the model vital to properly learn and apply it. In doing so, we hope to honor Dr Typaldos' memory while ensuring that new generations of FDM practitioners can easily reference a text with the core content of the model.

For years we have needed a quality text to accompany FDM teaching modules. Practitioners studying for their International Certificate exam have been directed to the fourth edition of Dr Typaldos' book as their primary study guide, but unfortunately, the rarity of that text today means that many are unable to obtain it. It is our aim that this text will serve as a new resource to accompany the instruction of both the European Fascial Distortion Model Association and the American Fascial Distortion Model Association. We also hope that it will be a suitable study guide for the International Certificate offered by member organizations of the Fascial Distortion Model Global Organization.

Todd Capistrant, Fairbanks, Alaska
Georg Harrer, Vienna, Austria
October 2020

ACKNOWLEDGMENTS

The completion of this project comes with a significant sensation of relief. We have been in desperate need of a text to accompany our FDM courses in the US, and I am extremely grateful to Dr Georg Harrer for the opportunity to collaborate on this project. Working through the manuscript, sharing ideas, and bantering via email has helped me learn more and given me a deeper understanding of the model. I am forever grateful for his expertise and ability to teach so effectively.

I would also like to thank Dr Thomas Pentzer for stepping forward to help with this complex project. His ability to craft grammatically correct sentences from the words I provided him is nothing short of miraculous.

Dr Gurkirat (Gary) Brar was instrumental in capturing the photos in this text. His skill with the camera, combined with his patience, allowed us to obtain the photos that will assist you while learning FDM.

I would like to acknowledge and thank Brandy Coltellaro for tolerating the time and energy that a project like this takes from family life. Without her amazing support and encouragement, a project like this could never have been successful. I am so grateful for all the things she took care of so that I could put the necessary energy into this work, and also for stepping outside her comfort zone and volunteering to be the model in the photos.

Finally, I would like to acknowledge the patients, without whom learning the FDM would not be possible. I am grateful that you have allowed us to join you on this journey to reduce pain, improve function, and restore movement.

Todd Capistrant

I feel the greatest gratitude for my mentor, the late Stephen Typaldos, who has changed my life with his discovery of the Fascial Distortion Model. Marge and John Kasten should also be mentioned here. Nobody has ever contributed more to spread the FDM for God's reward. Their unparalleled support as assistant and proofreader enabled Dr Typaldos to teach and publish, so without this support, the FDM would probably not have spread in these critical early days and the authors of this book would never have heard of it. I also have to thank the Vienna School of Osteopathy, where I was introduced to the FDM when Stephen Typaldos gave the first three day FDM Seminar in the world.

This book would not have been possible without the support of my wife Susanna, who gave me permission to participate in such an unprofitable undertaking as writing a book. I don't take this for granted.

Without the persistence and endurance of Andrew Stevenson, Mary Law, and all the kind and supportive people at Handspring, the book would not have been made.

Finally, I want to thank my father, Karl Harrer who many decades ago opened my eyes to the beauty and the importance of the connective tissue.

Georg Harrer

LIST OF ABBREVIATIONS

AACD	anterior ankle continuum distortion	**HVLA**	high-velocity, low-amplitude
ACL	anterior cruciate ligament	**IT**	iliotibial
ASIS	anterior superior iliac spine	**PSIS**	posterior superior iliac spine
CD(s)	continuum distortion(s)	**rFD(s)**	refolding distortion(s)
CTS	carpal tunnel syndrome	**ROM**	range of motion
CTLS	carpal tunnel-like syndrome	**SCM**	sternocleidomastoid muscle
CyD	cylinder distortion	**SCHTP**	supraclavicular herniated trigger point
DVT	deep vein thrombosis	**SI**	sacroiliac
EMG	electromyography	**TF**	tectonic fixation
FD(s)	folding distortion(s)	**TMJ**	temporomandibular joint
FDM	Fascial Distortion Model	**uFD(s)**	unfolding distortion(s)
HTP(s)	herniated trigger point(s)		

The Fascial Distortion Model (FDM) is a very specific concept. A few preliminary considerations may be helpful to achieve a better understanding of the innovation offered by the FDM.

General considerations with respect to medical concepts

Since the beginning of humanity, we have been accompanied by pain, weakness, and many other ailments. These issues are unlikely to have changed significantly over millennia. Physicians and healers throughout history strove to develop explanations for the illnesses and physical complaints of their contemporaries, and depending on the time and place, the cause of an ailment might be explained as an evil spell, God's punishment, an imbalance of the four humors, or bone marrow edema. Healers regarded their current explanations as "correct" and all previous and other explanations as at least obsolete, if not wholly wrong.

These explanations of the causes of illness are generally called "diagnoses" from ancient Greek "διαγνῶναι (diagnonai)," meaning "total insight" or "to comprehend something completely". Diagnoses or commonly shared understandings are beneficial tools to communicate, learn, teach, and develop treatment methods. The concept of diagnosis is ubiquitous: all styles of medicines – be they Western, Eastern, or ancient – use some form of diagnostic practice to guide their treatments. No matter how fundamentally different these diagnoses seem, in the end, they are applied to the same patients, the same diseases, and the same physiology.

Diagnosis

All diagnoses consist of these elements.

- **Etiology**, explaining the cause of the disease
- **Pathogenesis**, how the disease leads to the specific changes in the body
- Set of **symptoms** that the patient is expected to have
- Set of objective **findings**, which the physician is obliged to look for
- **Prognosis**, a natural course of the disease, with or without treatment
- **Treatment approach**, which is mainly based on the pathogenesis
- **Prophylaxis**, which is mainly based on the etiology

These elements may appear obvious, but we often overlook their transitory nature. All diagnoses are envisioned as a "true understanding" of the disease in the ancient Greek sense of the word, but the explanations may be replaced in a few decades by the next upcoming "truth". This process of explanations changing and being superseded is understood as scientific progress. The patient's complaints, however, remain unchanged over the ages.

Findings

Findings, a common basis for diagnoses, are collected by physicians following a given diagnostic pathway. They seem to be even more "real" than the diagnoses: an X-ray, a blood pressure reading, or an electrocardiogram are all objective findings, not subjective interpretations, and so they seem to represent the truth concerning the patient. But in a single patient, myriad findings are possible; far exceeding the capabilities of a physician in terms of time, financial resources, and cognitive capacity, and so all medical approaches are based on reduction to the essential findings. The specifics of this reduction are based on the current understanding of the disease more than on the disease itself. One could say the findings are what is left over when one ignores everything not regarded to be of interest, and as a result, the findings are only a very small part of the truth. A finding is not false, but due to the absence of all other ascertainable findings, it is not the complete or total truth representing the patient's condition. A finding may have more to do with the background of the physician than that of the patient: in other words, generally orthopedists take X-rays, internists order blood tests, and traditional Chinese doctors observe the tongue and feel the pulse. The patient's condition hardly influences this process.

Innovation

In general, new medical concepts evolve from older concepts. In the history of medicine, especially in Western allopathic medicine (which is what we usually understand as "medicine"), massive paradigm shifts are rare. Instead, progress is achieved step-by-step. Once there is an alpha-blocker, it is only a question of time before a beta-blocker is introduced, followed by a highly specific alpha-1-blocker, and so on. At no point in the development of these incremental changes is the underlying concept questioned.

There are, of course, exceptions. Examples include Robert Koch's infection theory, Sigmund Freud's psychoanalysis, or Edward Jenner's vaccination (more than a century before the first virus was discovered). These concepts do not represent incremental changes from prior concepts: they are major changes of paradigms; generally less appreciated by their contemporaries, but strongly valued by later generations.

Between 1992 and 1995, the US American physician Stephen P. Typaldos introduced an entirely new medical concept in several publications. He called this concept the **Fascial Distortion Model (FDM)**.

The Fascial Distortion Model (FDM) is an anatomical perspective in which injury and disease are considered to be comprised of one or more of six specific distortions in the body's connective tissue (Typaldos, 2002).

This statement is so clear and simple that the radical differences between this and other paradigms is not readily apparent to the majority of those exposed to it. Even Typaldos, with his medical background, had difficulties applying the FDM to all disorders, so he reduced its application to "... virtually every musculoskeletal injury (and many neurological and medical conditions as well) (Typaldos, 2002, p. 3)."

While the clinical application of the FDM historically focused on so-called "musculoskeletal" disorders, the number of indications outside this category grew within a few years. With the burgeoning list of indications, Typaldos struggled with determining the limits of this new concept. The situation was not unlike that of Robert Koch and his postulates, with regular discoveries of infectious agents as causes of conditions not previously considered to be infectious, like gastric ulceration and *H. pylori*, or cervical cancer and human papillomavirus (HPV). In the fourth edition of his FDM textbook, Typaldos (2002, p. 3) predicted "... perhaps the biggest impact of all will be on cardiology ..." even though most of the book focuses on "musculoskeletal" conditions.

While this book is intended to provide a framework for the contemporary application of the FDM in medicine, the authors will not attempt to define the limitations of the FDM itself.

Why fascia?

Stephen P. Typaldos was a doctor of osteopathic medicine and worked in many emergency departments around the USA. At no point in his career was he focused on "fascial research" or "fascial science." These fields of study barely existed in those days, and if a few physicians, anatomists, or other scientists took an interest in fascia, it was primarily academic rather than clinical.

Typaldos focused on his patients' descriptions of complaints, discussed treatment approaches with them, and observed their perception of these treatments. He was frustrated by his inability to match the patients' descriptions with any diagnoses in which he was trained. The location and types of complaints he observed in his patients had only one tissue in common that could reasonably explain the disorder: fascia. In addition, the patterns of pain followed pathways that could only be associated with fascial fibers. He undertook dissections in the pathology lab to look for muscles or other tissue missing in the anatomical textbooks, but his findings confirmed fascial fibers were the tissue involved.

Through his experiences in clinic and in the dissection lab, Typaldos understood fascia as a vast and important sensory organ that has exclusive access to information by measuring the tension of its fibrous web throughout the entire body.

Why distortion?

Typaldos struggled to define these fascial abnormalities to make targeted treatment possible.

Immediately he understood the importance of clear distinctions between these new diagnoses, which he called "distortions." Later, his definitions would prove valuable in teaching and research. Once a specific distortion is identified, a meaningful treatment, even a treatment that does not exist yet, can be imagined when the concepts of the FDM are applied to the patient's complaint.

Why only six distortions?

Between Spring 1991 and Fall 1992, Typaldos defined six different conditions, which, though interacting with each other, appeared to be distinct, reproducible entities. Typaldos, and later his students, continued to search for further distortions up to the present day, but additional distortions have yet to be identified. However, neither Typaldos, nor others who now work with the model, exclude the possibility of discovery of further distortions in future.

Why is it called the Fascial Distortion *Model?*

A model is a meaningful, comprehensible abbreviation of reality.

In natural science, there is no truth. Reality itself cannot be comprehended, because humans can only perceive what they are looking for, driven by their expectations, their senses and the tools they have available to them. Despite these limitations, humans tend to mistake their interpretation of reality with reality itself. In physics and other natural sciences, models are frequently used to help distill and codify data for ease of visualization and extrapolation. Models also provide a framework for the interpretation of novel data and are capable of evolving as more data is obtained.

It is important to realize that the FDM is not merely a kluge of diagnoses and techniques patched together. The FDM is a way of thinking as much as it is an approach to treatment.

On a supracellular level, form is defined by fascia. Without fascia, tissue is rather amorphous. Fascia defines the architecture in the body and guides the distribution of forces (van den Berg, 2017). In order to distribute forces, a three-dimensional layout of fibers and the liquid between them is essential. It seems reasonable to define an ideal form of fibrous arrangement for certain tasks, since the optimal transfer of forces requires an optimal arrangement of load-bearing structures. Unfortunately, given the complex multi-directional forces the human body is exposed to, and the limitations of visualization technologies, this ideal form cannot be visualized in nature. These limitations are not at all exclusive for fascia; they are intrinsic elements of all visualization strategies.

Triggerbands: twisted fascial bands

Parallel fibers are an ideal arrangement for the transmission of longitudinal forces. Within the Fascial Distortion Model (FDM), there is a type of fascia defined as "banded fascia" (Typaldos, 2002, p. 9). This type of fascia can be found in the entire body, wherever longitudinal forces have to be absorbed or created.

A **triggerband** is a pathology within this banded fascia (Fig. 3.1). Due to the parallel arrangement of the fibers, there is little resistance to shearing forces, that is, forces from oblique or transverse directions. These non-parallel forces are the cause of twists in the banded fascia.

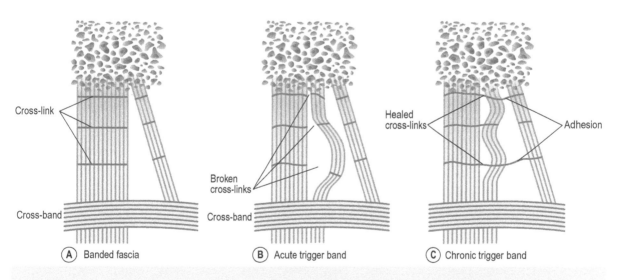

Cross-link

Cross-band

(A) Banded fascia

Broken cross-links

Cross-band

(B) Acute trigger band

Healed cross-links

Adhesion

(C) Chronic trigger band

FIGURE 3.1
Trigger bands (A) Banded fascia, (B) Acute trigger band, (C) Chronic trigger band.

It must be emphasized that the triggerband is a pathology. It occurs wherever unphysiologic forces hit the banded fascia, or wherever the banded fascia has lost its resilience due to other factors.

The physiologic behaviors of the twisted fibers are predictable. Fascial bands are exactly as long as they have to be. A twisted band will always be shorter than an untwisted band, and this shortening will lead to a limitation in range of motion (ROM). Furthermore, the sensory function of the fascia requires perfect alignment of the fibers to gain valid data, and so proprioception is inevitably altered along the fibers of a twisted fascial band.

Although the fibers of the banded fascia are infinite, the spread of a triggerband is limited. To understand this, we first need to clarify what we mean by defining fibers as "infinite". Fascial fibers can always be followed, but the current anatomical model defines borders where names change, e.g. the end of a tendon is defined by the beginning of a muscle. At the level of fascia, there is no muscle. The fascia ensheathes, surrounds, and shapes the muscle. The fibers pass through the muscle, which can be observed in advanced atrophy where the muscle looks more and more like a tendon. In the FDM, muscle is seen as a contractile tissue within the fascial construct. The same applies to bone: in the FDM, bone is understood as calcified banded fascia. The mineral composition differs, but the continuity of the fascial fibers is seamless throughout the bone. (This will be expanded on in the continuum distortion section see p. 8).

Although fascial fibers are continuous, the triggerband is limited either by bone or by crossing fascia. A triggerband is, by definition, an alteration of form in the banded fascia. Bone, with its mineral matrix, is form-stable, thus, the triggerband terminates where the fibers enter bone.

Under certain circumstances, the triggerband can enter or even pass through the bone. To allow this, the mineral matrix of the bone must alter its form accordingly, i.e. it must fracture. The fracture is an indispensable necessity for a triggerband to penetrate the bone, but it is rare. In general, the bone resists these forces, limiting the triggerband. Crossing fibers of other fascial bands also resist these forces, limiting the triggerband, similar to a hem limiting a tear in fabric. This does not mean the fibers have to twist and separate all the way from bone to bone or crossing fascia once a triggerband occurs, but it is possible.

Once the fascial band is untwisted, and the fibers are realigned, the triggerband no longer exists.

Herniated triggerpoints (HTPs): protrusion of tissue through a fascial plane

There is fascia that holds us together – banded fascia (see p. 5). There is also fascia that separates us. In the body, there are numerous cavities separated by fascial planes (Fig. 3.2A). The arrangement of collagen fibers is different in these planes, depending on the different tasks they are intended for. The separating layers also serve as gliding surfaces between the cavities. They vary in shape and size, from the spacious abdomen, to the smaller muscle compartment, to the even smaller subcutaneous fatty lobe; but all these fascial sheaths and pouches have orifices to allow important structures to pass into or out of the cavity (Fig. 3.2B). A cavity without these connections lacks continuity, a necessity for life and is therefore classified as pathologic, like cysts or abscesses. All cavities have individual pressures that vary depending on various factors (Fig. 3.2C). Under certain circumstances, pressures within one cavity may drive tissue from one side of the fascial plane separating two spaces into the other, often by passing through an orifice intended for something other than this tissue. Once this pathology occurs, it is addressed in the FDM as a **herniated triggerpoint** (HTP) (Fig. 3.2D).

The word "herniated" is an essential component of this term. The hernia as a surgical concept has many similarities to the HTP concept, but differs in its diagnostic criteria and the amount of offending tissue required. In surgery, where imaging is often used for diagnosis, a herniation must be large enough to be captured in the study for diagnosis: in HTPs, even small herniations are capable of disrupting normal physiology.

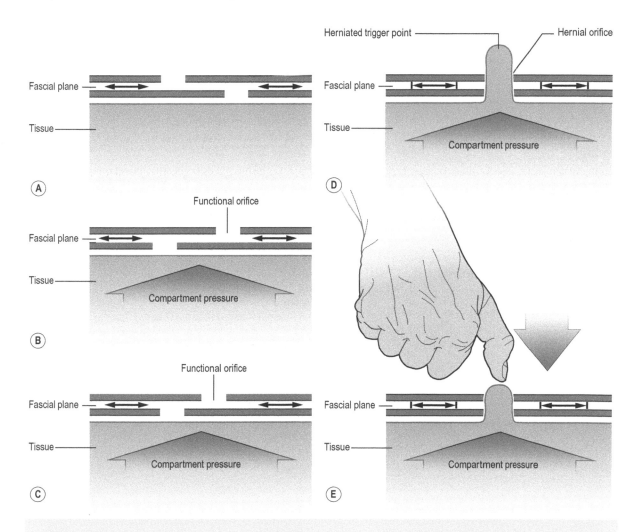

FIGURE 3.2
Herniated trigger point (HTP). (A) Body cavities separated by fascial planes. (B) Orifice in the cavity allowing passage of important structures. (C) Compartment pressure (D) HTP.

Many other schools of thought also use the term "triggerpoint." Most of these are systems of reflex points connected to some distant organ, or clinically defined zones that produce an alteration in a target organ, such as a muscle, once pressure or lidocaine is applied at these points. The connections between the "triggerpoint" and the target organ are presumed to be on a neural level. Aside from sharing a word, these concepts have nothing in common with the HTP concept and so are not discussed here.

As a general rule, it can be stated that compartmental pressures are higher in the deeper aspects of anatomy, and lower towards the superficial aspects of the body, which is why the majority of HTPs protrude from inside to outside. According to Typaldos (2002, p. 4), HTPs are more common on the trunk and less common on the extremities. However, they can and do occur throughout the entire body, wherever there is a fascial plane.

As a result of the protrusion, the fascial plane loses its capacity to glide (Fig. 3.2D). The herniated tissue holds it in place like a bolt, reducing the ROM of any body region dependent on the movement of the fascial plane for normal movement. Nociception and proprioception are also altered by the tension on the fascial fibers caused by the protrusion. Due to the specific architecture of the fascial plane, the extent of the alteration decreases with distance to the protrusion.

Once the protruded tissue is reduced (Fig. 3.2E), the altered fascial movement, nociception, and proprioception return to normal, and the HTP no longer exists.

Continuum distortions (CDs)

The transition between bone and fascial bands, such as ligaments or tendons and bone, is usually termed "insertion". Insertion derives from the Latin word "insero," the meaning of which pertains to inserting or implanting, much as a shoot is grafted onto the trunk of a tree (Pentzer, 2019).

In the FDM, the transition zone between bone and fascia is interpreted differently. Bone and ligament are not regarded as two discrete structures, but one continuous structure that merely differs in the number of osseous components (Harrer, 2017, p. 363), thus the fascial fibers form a seamless network throughout the body. In utero, mineral components are stored in sections of the fascia to prepare the embryo for later resistance to gravity and other forces. Breathing, for example, is not possible without form-stable structures around the lungs. This process continues for years until all zones of the fascia that require form and stability have enough osseous components to maintain that form under forces from random directions. At the same time, around other zones of fascia, minerals like calcium and phosphate remain in solution and are not used for osseous structures. These mineral-free zones are crucial necessities for later movement. The endoskeleton, called "continuum" in the FDM (Typaldos, 1995, p. 31), is a seamless organ of stability and mobility throughout the entire body.

Through the lens of FDM, bones do not exist as discrete entities: terms such as femur, radius, or vertebra are only used to define a region. The overriding characterization of bones as discrete entities may be because the mineral components of the fascial network remain long after soft tissue has decomposed, and so the continuous nature of the mineralized and unmineralized parts of the fascial network was unrealized and unappreciated until Typaldos developed the FDM.

In this continuum, there are also no ligaments. The banded fascia passes seamlessly through the mineralized zones, and wherever the mineralization starts and stops, banded fascia is named differently by the anatomists. In the FDM, these so-called ligaments are the non-mineralized zones of the continuum. Names like "anterior cruciate ligament" or "tibiotalar ligament" are again only communication tools for physicians, not a consideration of said ligaments as distinct entities.

Inside the mineralized zone (bone), continuous fascial fibers are crucial for stability. Minerals have little resistance to tension. Consider the building material known as steel-reinforced concrete: this durable material consists of two rather weak components: concrete, a mineral mixture which breaks immediately once minor traction or bending forces are applied, and steel, which in the form of rebar is not form-stable, allowing construction workers to bend sticks with their bare hands. However, once these two components are combined and the rebar is embedded in the concrete matrix, it is the strongest material humankind has ever invented for building. In the human skeleton, collagen fibers are the steel rebar, and calcium phosphate is the concrete.

Since embryological development is a never-ending story, and we change or refresh our tissues throughout our lives, mineral distribution in the continuum is never final. The transition zone between the mineralized zone (bone) and the non-mineralized zone (ligament) maintains the capability of mineralizing and demineralizing within minutes. When motion with multi-directional forces is demanded, the transition zone shifts into the ligamentous configuration, retaining minimal osseous components. When resting, minerals shift into the transition zone and form the osseous configuration. Due to entropy, mineral molecules in a liquid solution in the human body are always driven from a zone of high concentration to a zone of lower concentration. Energy-consuming cellular activity forces the minerals back into the bone when stimulated by stress and motion and consequently, the transition zone remains dynamic until death.

This phenomenon can be observed in imaging after long periods without forces applied to the transition zone. In the Intensive Care Unit, where patients are at rest for weeks or months, mineral components shift to the non-mineralized zones of the continuum (Fukuoka, et al, cited in Harrer, 2017, p. 364), leading to osteoporosis in the mineralized zone and ossification, such as osteophytes or myositis ossificans, in the non-mineralized zones. These symptoms are not seen as specific diagnoses in the FDM, but as reversible exaggerations of physiology under unnatural conditions.

The phenomenon of minerals shifting in the transition zone is only useful when the entire zone in one location shifts to either of the two configurations (osseous or ligamentous). If some fibers of the transition zone mineralize (osseous configuration) and other fibers within the same transition zone demineralize (ligamentous configuration), the transition zone is not functional. This is known as a **continuum distortion** (CD) (Fig. 3.3). CDs can be divided into two subtypes, **inverted** and **everted** (discussed later in the treatment section, see p. 41).

The etiology of this maldistribution of transition zone minerals is not entirely clear. The osseous configuration is not well-suited for handling multi-directional forces and the application of multi-directional forces to the transition zone in the osseous configuration is one of the possible mechanisms of injury. Trauma is by no means the sole cause of CDs, however, and in some cases, a metabolic origin is more likely.

CDs can only be understood using the continuum model. Envisioning bones and ligaments as distinct entities, as in the current anatomical model, counteracts this process of understanding. As medical professionals are trained with this current anatomical "parts" model, it can be difficult for them to adapt to the continuum

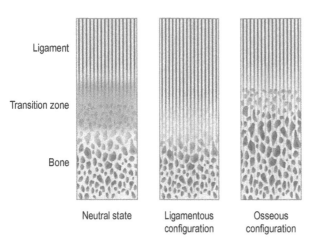

Ligament

Transition zone

Bone

Neutral state   Ligamentous configuration   Osseous configuration   Continuum distortion

FIGURE 3.3
Functional and dysfunctional configurations within the continuum.
(A) The transition zone has the ability to shift its components. (B) The transition zone becomes demineralized (ligamentous configuration). (C) The transition zone becomes mineralized (osseous configuration). (D) Both configurations within the same transition zone mean it is not functional and therefore is a pathology (**continuum distortion**, CD).

theory, and people without medical training usually have fewer problems understanding the theory.

As with all fascial distortions, a CD is reversible. Once the transition zone has returned to normal, it can shift between its two physiologic configurations (osseous and ligamentous) and the CD no longer exists.

Folding distortions (FDs)

There is a fascial arrangement in the body which is responsible for safe and guided movement. In general, joint stability is seen as an effect of muscle action, controlled by proprioception and reflexes. However, stable movement is also possible when performed passively, without muscular input. Under the influence of muscle-relaxing drugs, such as those used in general anesthesia, a joint can be moved again and again without dislocation of its components. There must be another underlying stability factor, one that is only augmented by muscle action. In the FDM, this specific fascial arrangement is envisioned as folding fascia (Fig. 3.4). This arrangement allows the fascia to repeatedly unfold and refold in the same manner without wear or resistance. In a tubular arrangement, as can be assumed around joints, the mechanism of folding fascia can be understood through the analogy

of a concertina or accordion. In planes, such as interosseous membranes or intermuscular septa, a folded paper roadmap analogy is more helpful to understand the mechanism.

Dissecting distortions

The anatomical perspective applied in the FDM does not contain separate entities or parts. Terms like "the capsule" do not apply to the location of folding fascia. Fascial anatomy is understood as continuous and functional. Regional distribution of a feature such as folding fascia is a functional attribute, independent of any specific part of the body, and so cannot be displayed in dissection. Dissection is a tool developed for the current anatomical model. All dissections produce artifacts secondary to the goals and ideas of the dissector.

As long as the natural folds of the folding fascia are present (Fig. 3.4A), all movement is reversible, with the folds guiding everything back to its proper place, even after numerous repetitions (Fig. 3.4B, C).

The folding fascia is most stable in the middle of the range between unfolding and refolding. As the folding fascia moves to either end of this range, fascial wrinkles disappear. When the moving zone is completely distracted (Fig. 3.4D) or compressed, it becomes prone to distortion (Fig. 3.4E). In general, additional forces are involved, either from muscle contraction or external sources. Fascial distortion can only occur when the folding fascia is in either of its two vulnerable configurations (traction or compression) when forces act upon the fascia.

There are therefore two subtypes of FD: **unfolding distortion** (uFD) and **refolding distortion** (rFD) depending on the arrangement that caused the injury. These distortions require different treatment strategies, which will be discussed in the treatment chapters.

As with all fascial distortions, FDs are reversible. Once fascia regains its three-dimensional shape, its folding ability is restored (Fig. 3.4F), and the FD no longer exists.

Cylinder distortions (CyDs)

Another type of fascia is understood to hold everything in place: the fascia found between all structures, such as muscles, vessels, or skin. Typaldos termed this the "superficial fascia" (Typaldos 2002, p. 47), even though it is not only found in the superficial layers of the body.

The key aspect of this fascial arrangement is its cylindrical layout of fibers. A specimen of subcutaneous fascia studied under a microscope does not show a preferred direction of fibers: instead the fibers crisscross in all directions, leading to the conclusion that it is a random arrangement, not unlike a handful of spaghetti dropped to the ground. In the FDM, however, this microscopic image is interpreted differently: the fact that we can never identify the end of a fiber in these specimens means the term "fibers"(plural) is hypothetical. To use an

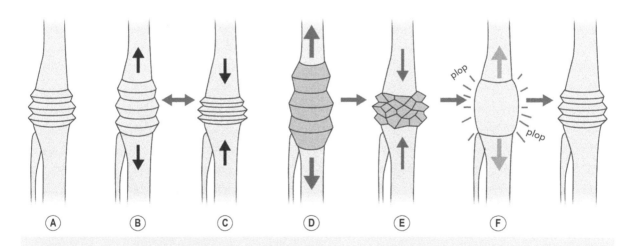

FIGURE 3.4
Folding distortion (FD). (A) When folding fascia maintains its natural folds, all movement is reversible, even after numerous repetitions (B, C). When the moving zone is completely distracted (D) or compressed, it becomes prone to distortion (E). Once the fascia regains its three-dimensional shape, the folding ability of the fascia is restored (F).

analogy: when we look at a small area of a ball of wool, we might get the impression of multiple random strands of yarn, but if we look more closely we will find a single fiber in a particular, self-similar arrangement. The architecture of this ball of wool can be understood as a system of recursive circles of a single wool fiber.

In the human body, which is more cylindrical than spherical, the concentric circles in the ball of wool analogy become coils, comprising complex

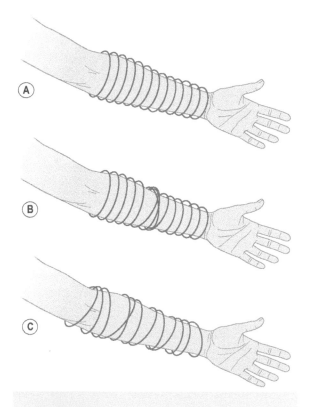

FIGURE 3.5
Cylinder distortion (CyD) (A) To allow multi-directional flexibility and elasticity, cylinder coils must be able to move freely and absorb forces multi-directionally. If the cylinder arrangement becomes entangled, we see CyD (B, C).

cylinders. These cylinders explain the ability of the connective tissue to counteract multi-directional forces with the same stability. When skin is pulled away from the body, it snaps back into its normal position as soon as the applied force is terminated. In the FDM, cylindrical fascia is understood as a shock absorbing system, holding everything in place even under strong or repetitive forces, in all regions and layers of the body. In order to allow this multi-directional flexibility and elasticity, the coils of the cylinders must be able to move freely without obstructing each other, as forces have to be absorbed multi-directionally by a synergetic system of interwoven cylinders (Fig. 3.5A).

Once the coils of this cylindrical arrangement become entangled, we see a specific pathology called cylinder distortion (CyD) (Fig. 3.5B). Due to the presence of cylindrical fascia all over the body, this distortion can occur anywhere in the body.

As with all fascial distortions, CyD is reversible. Once the entangled coils are separated, and the cylinders can move freely without mutual obstruction, CyD no longer exists.

Tectonic fixations (TFs)

Fascia has the ability to glide. All human joints, whether they are saddle joints or ball-and-socket joints, are considered sliding bearings. There are no ball or roller bearings, nor do we find needle bearings as in a compass. Anatomists claim certain components must be present for a structure to be addressed as a joint, such as capsule, or cartilage. These criteria are an artifact of the anatomist and do not fully appreciate the functionality of all moving areas.

All moving areas follow the same principle. The scapulothoracic joint moves just as effectively as the glenohumeral, without capsule or cartilage.

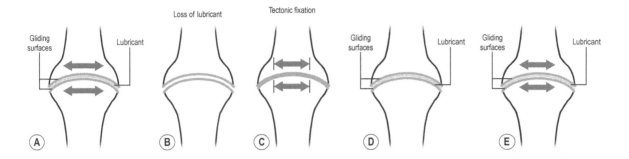

FIGURE 3.6
Tectonic fixation (TF). A joint has two corresponding surfaces and a layer of fluid in between (A). If movement ceases and fluid stops being produced, fascial surfaces lose their ability to glide, and become stiff (B) resulting in TF (C). Once the lubricant fluid layer is restored (D), TF is reversed (E).

The essential components of a sliding bearing or joint are the same in nature as in engineering: two corresponding surfaces and a layer of fluid between them (Fig. 3.6A). Neither the fluid layer nor the surfaces are more important than the other; both are crucial. This principle applies to the fascia around joints as much as it applies to layers of fascia in the back. Whether it is located near a joint or not, fascia must glide in different ways to make movement possible.

Lubricant fluid is produced in response to demand by the body (van den Berg, 2017, p. 39). Movement and applied forces stimulate its production: as long as we move, we produce this lubricant. Once fluid production is halted due to cessation of movement, the fascial surfaces lose their ability to glide, and stiffness will be observed (Fig. 3.6B). In the FDM, the term for this pathology is **tectonic fixation** (TF) (Fig. 3.6C).

As with all fascial distortions, TF is reversible. Once the lubricant fluid layer is restored between the sliding bearings (Fig. 3.6D), the TF no longer exists (Fig. 3.6E).

Natural progression of fascial distortions

The concept of fascial distortions leads to a few questions. How did humankind cope with fascial distortions in the past? Who fixed these fascial distortions before the FDM was developed?

When we assume that there are inherent, natural healing mechanisms, like the immune system in infection theory, we have to compare our treatment results with this natural progression. If our treatments prolong the symptoms or have poorer outcomes than natural progression, we are obliged to change our strategies. Therefore, we have to study the interaction between our body's repair mechanisms and the fascial distortions before commencing treatment.

Triggerbands

Triggerbands start acute and tend to become chronic.

This sounds like a platitude and seems to apply to any injury or illness, but in the FDM, the terms "chronic" and "acute" apply exclusively to the triggerband: the other five fascial distortions cannot become chronic, and the notions of acute or chronic do not apply.

Chronicity in the FDM

The word chronicity derives from the ancient Greek word Χρόνος describing the measurable aspect of time. Different to Καιρός, ancient Greek for the right moment, the best point of time for an action to be taken, Χρόνος is the quantity of time, such as seconds, years, or centuries. In general, chronicity is defined as the self-perpetuation of a condition, even after elimination of the original noxious agent. Other definitions of chronicity define acute as localized and responsive to treatment, while chronic is non-localized and less or unresponsive to treatment. All these phenomena are widely observed, but the terms are only descriptive. Lacking a pathophysiological model, chronicity is linked to time. As a discrete mechanism, how the passage of time determines responsiveness to treatment is unknown.

A triggerband is a twisted fascial band. As described above, the band has multiple parallel longitudinal fibers with a low number of cross-links. The fibers themselves are unlimited, but the architectural zone in which a triggerband can occur is finite. The features of the triggerband are the separation of longitudinal fibers plus a twist, changing the two-dimensional arrangement of the banded fascia into a three-dimensional one.

Once present, the triggerband can develop in several ways:

1. The triggerband heals slowly on its own via inherent wound healing mechanisms. This complex strategy of organisms is a co-operation of various humoral and cellular activities, including macrophage and fibroblast activity, fibrin deposition, hyperemia, swelling, and so on. The ability to heal a wound is essential for any higher organism. The disadvantages of this course are the slow speed and the likelihood of a poor outcome quality if the circumstances during the healing process are suboptimal.

2. The triggerband is immediately repaired by a measure that restores the natural arrangement of the fascial band. This option might be considered utopian, but it is the only desirable outcome, once we envision the condition as a twisted fascial band.

3. The triggerband becomes chronic. We do not fully understand the pathophysiology of chronicity; nevertheless, this is the least desirable outcome because the triggerband is less likely to resolve than in the other three options.

4. The triggerband remains acute. This does not sound appealing on the first glimpse, but there are far better chances to reach a perfect result, *restitutio ad integrum*, once circumstances improve or an adequate treatment is applied.

Considering these four options, chronicity seems to be the most mysterious and least desirable. The FDM offers a specific pathophysiological definition for chronicity, which explains the altered response to treatment (Fig. 3.1).

During the healing process, fibroblasts reconnect the separated fibers by enforcing the initial fibrin attachments with collagen fibers. Some of the collagen fibers reunite the separated longitudinal fibers. Others connect the fibers to random neighboring fascial bands. In the long history of life, movement and load guided the fibroblasts. In nature, rest is a limited option. Hence, wound healing is guided by motion and load. Exclusively fascial structures that move together should heal together. Those who move separately not only should not heal together, they must not heal together. If they do so, future motion will be obstructed by adhesion.

In common therapeutic strategies that incorporate rest as a major component, the fibroblasts, deprived of information, connect everything in the vicinity of the separated fibers. A long and tedious process is needed after that to counteract these adhesions, called rehabilitation. Resting and immobilization create the demand for later rehabilitation. Hence resting strategies are not considered useful in the FDM.

The "Ziploc™" analogy for the triggerband applies here. A bunch of Ziploc bags can be moved in any direction, gliding on each other, all remaining closed during this maneuver, but once attached to each other by glue or suture, the bags will rip each other open when forced to move. This explains why the initial injury is no longer needed to propagate and spread the condition.

In the FDM, "acute" is a triggerband without adhesions and "chronic" is a triggerband with adhesions. This means chronicity is determined by the state of the tissue, not by the time elapsed. Different from the time-theory, this perspective opens many new options. The conduct of time is unchangeable. Adhesions can be broken at any point. Lysis of adhesions will change a chronic triggerband into an acute triggerband, and resting does the opposite.

Heat applied to the tissue in resting position speeds up the process of becoming chronic, since it accelerates the ability of fibroblasts to synthesize collagen and amplifies the supply of protein and energy. Ordinarily, this may be considered beneficial, but it lacks the crucial simultaneous information of movement and load. In nature, tissue only becomes

warmer when it is working, and fibroblasts are not prepared for thermal therapy without movement.

The triggerband starts acute and inclines to become chronic. Resting, immobilization, and heat amplify this process.

Herniated triggerpoints (HTPs)

HTPs have a sudden onset and are permanent.

The HTP comes into existence at the very moment tissue protrudes through the fascial plane. If more tissue protrudes later, it might aggravate the HTP, but the initial onset is sudden.

Without reduction, the HTP is permanent. Due to the ongoing pressure gradient, without an option to produce negative pressure (suction) inside the body, the herniation is doomed to remain unchanged until reduced by external pressure. The prognosis without treatment is poor.

It has to be emphasized that there are no chronic HTPs. As stated above, chronicity is an exclusive feature of the triggerband. Due to the absence of a wound, there is no potential for adhesions. As a ramification of this, an HTP always has the same prognosis and the likelihood of a successful reduction is the same, no matter how long the HTP has existed.

Continuum distortions (CDs)

CDs develop suddenly and have the ability to shift back to normal.

Once the transition zone between the mineralized and non-mineralized zone distorts, causing osseous and ligamentous configuration at the same time in one spot, the transition zone can no longer shift between its two physiologic configurations. If cellular metabolic activities are able to restore calcium distribution to normal, the prognosis is good, in that this process leads to a *restitutio ad integrum* with calcium distribution in the transition zone restored to a normal physiologic arrangement. However, in some individuals, this restoration does not happen, and the CD remains. The mechanisms behind this phenomenon are currently unclear. Movement seems to facilitate restoration, but even in very active people, a CD may persist for a long time.

Because there is no wound involved in the pathophysiology of CDs, there is no wound healing, no fibroblast activity, and hence no chronic CDs. As a result, the likelihood of a successful restoration of the transition zone is the same no matter how long the CD has existed.

Folding distortions (FDs)

FDs have a sudden onset and are permanent.

FDs occur the instant a movement distorts the folding fascia. From this moment, the FD is present and will remain unchanged until refolded to the normal arrangement. Since various forces are applied to the body by different activities, the corrective vector of force may be introduced by chance. The more a person with an FD engages in different activities, the higher the chance for a "lucky draw" of force combinations that restore the folds of the folding fascia. Resting reduces this probability. If the vector that caused the FD is unusual, either in direction or in amplitude, there is a high chance that the FD will persists for many years, if not become permanent. This does not influence the likelihood of successful treatment.

Because there is no wound involved in the pathophysiology of FDs, there is no wound healing, no fibroblast activity, and hence no adhesions and no chronic FDs. The likelihood of success of a measure to restore the natural folds is the same no matter how long the FD has existed.

Cylinder distortions (CyDs)

CyDs have a sudden onset and an almost unpredictable outcome.

Cylinder distortions (CyDs) are defined as the entangling of the cylindrical coils of the cylindrical fascia. In general, the symptoms arise suddenly, and the cause remains unclear in many cases. The geometry of a CyD is already complex when we imagine one single coil of cylindrical fascia becoming entangled. Once multiple interwoven coils entangle, the complexity exceeds any calculability, and the prognosis is not predictable. The number and severity of complaints are also not predictive. Some CyDs are fixed easily; others stubbornly resist treatment. Nevertheless, CyDs cannot become chronic since they do not develop adhesions.

Tectonic fixations (TFs)

TFs develop gradually, caused by other fascial distortions that reduce motion of the affected region. The prognosis is linked to the outcome of the underlying distortions.

TFs never develop independently of other distortions; they develop gradually due to a regional lack of movement. One or more of the other five fascial distortions cause an ongoing loss of mobility in the affected region, leading to a significant reduction of lubricant fluid. TFs may occur in joints with cartilage and synovial fluid, as well as in gliding tissue without cartilage, anywhere the amount of extracellular fluid is reduced. The lack of fluid universally leads to progressive stiffness. This stiffness terminates once the fluid layer is restored, once the underlying fascial distortions are no longer present.

It has to be emphasized that in many therapeutic concepts in physiotherapy, osteopathy, chiropractic, and other fields, mobility is understood as a goal of supreme importance. The slogan "life is motion" is very common. TFs are considered a considerable threat by members of these professions. In nature, this does not apply. Stability and durability are crucial; mobility is nice, so long as stability and durability are present. In the wilderness, a stiff and resilient knee is always preferable to a mobile but non-resilient one. With this in mind, TFs should not be perceived as worse than the other five distortions, and in some cases, might even be lifesaving for the individual. Even in modern societies with healthcare systems, some patients are happy once their ankle is finally stiff so long as it is also resilient.

TFs do not involve wounds or any discontinuity, and so there is no wound healing, no adhesions, and TFs cannot become chronic. Due to the progressive nature of TFs, the effort to restore mobility increases with the amount of stiffness, not with the amount of time elapsed since the onset.

In the FDM, a complex patient's history can be seen as an intricately braided rope. Once teased apart, the stories are easier to comprehend.

Introduction to diagnostics according to the Fascial Distortion Model (FDM)

There is no such thing as "fascial therapy." For "fascial therapy" to exist, "non-fascial therapy" would also need to exist, but due to its omnipresence in the body, all therapeutic approaches will influence the fascia. Massage therapy, for instance, is focused on treating muscles, but in fact, massage therapists treat their patients. With external manual techniques, no tissue can be treated in isolation. The skin is affected by external treatment, as are blood vessels, nerves, the periosteum, and so on. The only difference is what the individual therapists envision according to their paradigms. Similarly, muscle without its ensheathing fascia is a formless jelly, so "muscle training" in a gym can only be applied via fascia. All connections between the muscle and the outside world are fascial; all surgical procedures are bound to open fascial cavities and alter fascial continuity; all pharmaceutical treatment will involve fascia even though the pharmacological target might be the brain or the kidney. Drugs dissolve in the body's fluids and disperse through all tissues, and so all drugs might affect fascia, even though that effect is not their primary purpose. For example, a patient receiving a quinolone antibiotic for cystitis might end up with a ruptured Achilles tendon, a rare but well-known side effect of this drug.

Since there is no "non-fascial therapy," the term "fascial therapy" does not make sense: there is only treatment for fascial pathologies. As the pathology of the fascia is very specific, the treatment also has to be specific. This is by no means a quality unique to fascia: any dermatologist will admit that there is no treatment for skin in its general state of being, only for specific skin disorders. Diagnosis of a specific fascial disorder is crucial before considering any treatment for fascial distortion.

A few terms will be discussed in this chapter in order to gain a better understanding of diagnostic systems. Terms like "diagnosis" or "finding" are familiar to medically-trained people and further explanation may seem unnecessary; however, although these terms are used frequently in medical training, they are seldom explained.

Diagnosis

Diagnosis (ancient Greek "διαγνῶναι" [diagnonai]) means total insight. This suggests that there is a "real, true diagnosis" and all other diagnoses are therefore false. The term also suggests that diagnoses are distinct entities, like animals or persons, and this is how they are taught in medical schools. Medical students learn diagnoses like biologists learn animal species: "hemorrhagic disorders" and "autoimmune disease" are classifications just as "vertebrates" or "artiodactyla" are. But there is a fundamental difference. Animals like giraffes or sheep (both artiodactyla) exist; they were around long before the biologists that classify them. Animals *can* be described, but they do not *need* to be: they are real entities with or without our descriptions of them. Diagnoses are different, in that they are concepts: they only exist in the mind of physicians of the same "tribe," as collective theories shared by all medical staff within the same medical system.

This is not in any way a criticism. Collective visualizations and theories are necessary to co-operate, research, learn, and teach. Innumerable medical concepts in different parts of the world over millennia have been based on the collective imagination of diagnoses. For thousands of years, Chinese physicians categorized diagnoses according to five elements (wood, fire, earth, metal, and water) and in that school of thought, their patients suffered from a lack of water or too much earth. In Europe, humorism was the dominant model for thousands of years, in which medical diagnoses were based on a mismatch of the four humors (yellow bile, black bile, blood, and phlegm) and so patients were diagnosed as suffering from a lack of black bile or too much phlegm. All universities agreed on this, and libraries were full of books that dealt with the details of this concept. So over time and geography, diagnoses change, but the complaints remain the same. Back pain is not classical, medieval, or contemporary; European or Chinese. Back pain is always the same; only the medical perspectives change. Chinese people do not have different coughs to Europeans, only differently trained doctors.

This differentiation between complaints and diagnoses is very important when dealing with diagnostic systems. Nobody suffers from arthritis, joint overuse, or fascial distortions: people suffer from knee pain when going downstairs. The terms applied to knee pain are only medical interpretations of the patient's experience.

Medicine is not a natural science, in the sense that it is not about gaining insight like the field of physics; it is about justifying action. Again, these observations are not intended as criticism, but they are necessary to understand how diagnostic systems work. A diagnostic algorithm is not designed to find the truth, as many physicians think. It is designed to find the most suitable categorization available in the current medical system at this point in time. For example, it is likely that in 2020, we will observe a massive increase in "burnout syndrome" because burnout syndrome was classified as a diagnosis by the WHO in 2019.

On the other hand, we might observe a significant drop in anxiety, chronic fatigue, and depression because patients previously diagnosed with these disorders will now be categorized instead as suffering burnout syndrome, although their symptoms have not changed. In other eras, the diagnosis would have been "neurasthenia" (Beard, 1869) or "faith deficiency," treated with ice water baths or prayers, according to the fashion of the day.

Fascial distortions are also diagnoses, i.e. collective visualizations shared by all who apply the FDM.

Medical diagnoses are continually changing. Each new interpretation will change the diagnosis and allow new treatments which were impossible before. The identification of *H. pylori* as a cause of gastric ulcers is a good example of this kind of development. When infection theory, which had been around since 1876, was applied to this specific disorder in the 1980s, it revolutionized the medical approach to stomach ulcer treatment, seemingly overnight. The treatment itself, a very cheap antibiotic that had been around for decades, could not have been utilized before infection theory was applied to stomach ulcers, but following this change of paradigm, worldwide mortality rates for gastric cancer dropped significantly, not because of new technology, but because of the new model. One should keep in mind that, like other current diagnoses, *H. Pylori* is not the *true* cause of stomach ulcer; it is the *contemporary* cause of stomach ulcer and no doubt it will be replaced by future theories with better outcomes.

Findings

People might say, "Maybe a diagnosis is a collective theory, but an objective finding is 'true,' as it is 'objective'." Findings, in the medical sense, are clinical observations related to physical examination or laboratory testing. This does not sound like "truth."

The following definition is preferable: "A finding is the remnant of all observable features once an observer ignores everything he/she considers to be irrelevant."

Again, this is not a criticism. The entirety of all observable, measurable features of a patient is overwhelmingly large and cannot be gathered, documented, or comprehended. Technological, financial, cognitive, and many other limitations, such as urgency, force the clinician to ignore information that has no perceived relevance or associated meaning in the immediate context. Anyone who claims to "look at the entire patient" overestimates his/her capabilities. This approach would cost a fortune and would maybe consume the entire lifetime of the patient and the observer. It would include ECG, EEG, colonoscopy, perimetry, speech and gait analysis, spirometry, checking the tongue for coating, scintigram, PET scan, genome sequencing, audiogram, and even tasting the urine. Nobody can cope with this volume of information. The human brain is more of a data filter than a data collector and selects information based on relevance, to distinguish between what is important and what is unimportant. We mean to exclude the irrelevant and focus on the relevant. But how do we determine relevance? Who has the time and resources to compare all the possible features in terms of relevance? Generally, we ignore what our teachers told us to ignore, hence Chinese physicians check the tongue for coating, orthopedists take X-rays, and cardiologists interpret ECGs. Through the repeated application of their respective paradigms, each conclude that their choice is the most relevant.

Radiography is an excellent example of this reductive approach. Wilhelm Conrad Roentgen introduced his X-ray machine in 1895, providing physicians with a revolutionary method of evaluation. Before X-rays, all patients were visible: every observer could see the same aspects. Roentgen's machine made patients invisible. For the first time in history, physicians could look through their patients. The only material that defied invisibility was what could be seen on the X-rays (mainly air, calcium and water). Begging lenience from radiologists for over-simplification, on X-ray images, air is black, water is grey, and calcium is white and in principle, this is the basis of radiology. The crucial question is, why do we declare the truth is found in an artificial image where everything except water and calcium has been made invisible? Why do we look for the "truth" in the remaining 10% (water and calcium) and not in the 90% of tissue that has been made invisible?

What to look for? What to ignore?

All diagnostic strategies face similar challenges. It is a common pitfall that the purpose of diagnostics is to find out "what the patient really has." This is an entirely unscientific approach, and due to the absence of a referee, doomed to fail. The only valid questions are: "Does the patient have what the clinician thinks they have?" and "is there a test to find out?" Unfortunately, all tests are, to some extent, incorrect.

There are always four possibilities:

Suspect positive – Test shows positive (+/+)

Suspect positive – Test shows negative (+/-)

Suspect negative – Test shows positive (-/+)

Suspect negative – Test shows negative (-/-)

If these four possibilities were applied to four quarters of a dartboard, darts might deviate to one side or the other, as if magnets were influencing the flight of the dart. These magnets are "sensitivity" and "specificity." Some tests generate false positives: these tests are too sensitive. Some tests generate false negatives: these tests are too specific. In principle, this is the basis of diagnostics. Everybody wants a test that is 100% accurate, but there is no such test available for humans. Any test is limited by costs, time, technology, the involvement of human beings interpreting data, and many other factors. Moreover, the degree of sensitivity of a test can only be measured once there is a more sensitive test available for comparison. The same applies to specificity. At any point in time, the most advanced test is the benchmark, doomed to be replaced by a more sensitive or more specific test in the future.

Apart from sensitivity and specificity, all tests need another feature to justify their application: a test must be reproducible, that is to say that when ten radiologists interpret the same image, all ten should come exactly to the same diagnosis. This is unlikely to happen. There are two equally good outcomes: either all ten say the patient has a positive diagnosis, or all ten say the patient has a negative diagnosis. A poor outcome would be if five radiologists say the patient has a positive result, and five give a negative result. Fortunately, this is rare in radiology. In other diagnostic approaches like palpation, however, this 50/50 split is a common outcome. Flipping a coin would have the same value, but looks less professional. The term for this reproducibility is "**inter-rater reliability**."

Inter-rater reliability is easy to measure with a sample group of testers with standardized training, using the same technology or method and asked the same question. Some strategies have almost 99% inter-rater reliability; some others, far less. There are statistical methods to measure inter-rater reliability: the unit of measurement is $\varkappa$ (kappa, the Greek letter k). In general, a diagnostic approach with a high $\varkappa$-value is preferred. Many clinicians still use palpation for other reasons, even though there is strong evidence that the $\varkappa$-value is very poor.

Inter-rater reliability is an independent feature, not related to sensitivity, specificity, or relevance. Pigeons, for example, have (after two weeks of training) the same results in the detection of early breast cancer in mammography as radiologists (Levenson, 2015).

Another challenge is selecting the most appropriate diagnostic tool. In other words, what should we ignore (relevance)? A diagnostic method like ECG, even though showing high sensitivity, specificity, and inter-rater reliability for cardiac arrhythmias, is a poor choice to determine whether a patient has onychomycosis. In the majority of cases, relevance or its absence seems obvious. However, in some cases, it is not only not obvious; it is quite the opposite. Relevance is hard to measure, requiring comparison of large clinical cohorts. In order to determine the relevance of a diagnostic procedure, different and measurable treatment approaches are required, chosen according to the diagnostic algorithm. When a diagnostic algorithm enables us to differentiate fifteen different types of conjunctivitis, yet treatment for all fifteen is silver-nitrate eye drops (as was the case in the 1940s), the relevance of a differential diagnosis is hard to measure. In the presence of more specific treatments available 50 years later, the same diagnostic algorithm becomes more meaningful.

In many cases, relevance is determined by trends and the teacher's opinion, rather than on scientific evidence. For example, there is strong evidence that imaging strategies have no relevance in lower back pain, but nevertheless, imaging strategies are still the number one diagnostic tool in lower back pain in many countries (Maher, Underwood, and Buchbinder, 2017, Chou et al., 2009, Jensen et al., 1994). The number and depth of forehead skin wrinkles is a very strong indicator for the risk of early death from a cardiovascular incident and the significance of the wrinkles seems to be far higher than that of cholesterol level, ECG, and blood pressure, as demonstrated by Esquirol, et al. (2018), but despite this data, physicians adhere to their old predictors, even though they might be less reliable.

The considerations outlined above are no more important to the FDM than to any other medical approach, but the limitations of FDM diagnostics, like other diagnostic models, should be kept in mind. In the following chapters, common contemporary approaches for diagnosing fascial distortions will be discussed. If another diagnostic approach looks more promising than current methods, one should be able to determine the benefit of the new approach. Is its benefit sensitivity, specificity, inter-rater reliability, relevance, cost, or something else? The benefit to patient care should be specified before the current algorithms are questioned. Fashion or the teacher's opinion are weak arguments for changing the plan.

The fascial system is arguably the largest sensory organ of the body. (Some say the skin is larger, but it is hard to prove). Most proprioceptors and nociceptors are located in the fascia and the majority of the nervous system is dedicated to this inner sense. When we look at a cross-section of the spinal cord, half of the fibers are afferent. All these axons conduct information about pain, tension, position, and other internal qualities. It is the first sense that develops *in utero*. The embryo knows little about the exterior world but is already gathering information about its own limbs. Inability to receive information about position, strength, and tension is perhaps the worst disability, similar to tetraplegia, and removing the individual's ability to do anything purposefully. The case of the British butcher, Ian Waterman, who lost almost his entire proprioception within a few days is well described in *Living without Touch and Proprioception*, by Cole and Oppenheimer (2005, pp. 85–97).

Despite its importance, proprioception was not recognized for over two thousand years. Aristotle (384–322 BC) defined the five senses as sight, hearing, taste, smell, and touch and strictly excluded the future discovery of other senses. Though pain and perception of our own body were not included in these senses, Aristotle's theory was passed on for over two thousand years virtually unquestioned. In his 1833 publication, *The Hand*, Charles Bell (1774–1842), a Scottish physician known for first describing Bell's palsy, was the first to suggest a sixth sense, an inner sense for position and tension. Bell was the first in the long history of science to discover this scientific gap. It took another seventy-three years until Charles Scott Sherrington (1857–1952), the British physician and founder of neurophysiology, defined the terms "proprioception" and "nociception" in his book *The Integrative Action of the Nervous System* and introduced this "new" sensory organ to the scientific world in 1906.

The sensors of this inner sense of proprioception and nociception, all located in fascia, gather supreme information about the condition of fascia. This vast sensory organ is the basis for diagnostics in the FDM. The skin is, according to many authors, envisioned as an organ of its own and is equipped with a high density of nociceptors.

All concepts of subdivision of the body, especially traditional anatomy, take some issue with fascia. The concepts of organs, such as kidney, brain, or liver, originated in the early 19th century. Carl Rokitansky (1804–1878) was the leading pioneer in this field of "organ pathology." Before that, organs were not seen as entities of importance, but in the age of the industrial revolution, "parts" were a common analogy. The hype about organs in medicine was short-lived: by the second half of the 19th century, cellular pathology had replaced organ pathology. Later in the 20th and 21st centuries, genetic, epigenetic, and molecular pathology reduced the need for subdivisions of the human body. Even though organ pathology played only a brief role in medical history, the idea is still dominant because medical specialties are identified with it, i.e. there are heart doctors, lung doctors, and skin doctors, which suggests the existence of heart, lungs, and skin. On the level of fascia, there are no organs, only fiber arrangements, and embedded liquid and minerals, so from a fascial perspective, the dermis is a special arrangement of superficial fascia. Even in the skin, nociceptors are embedded in fascial fibers and proprioceptors, like the Ruffini corpuscles, are exclusively embedded in fascia. Since all proprioceptors, and the majority of nociceptors, are mechanoreceptors, they measure the mechanics of fascia. The three-dimensional sense of position and tension is based on the measurement of the movement of fascial fibers. Once the deformation has exceeded a certain threshold, nociceptors detect this deformation, and we feel pain.

The basis of FDM diagnostics is the hypothesis that nociception and proprioception are the supreme sources of information concerning the shape of fascia. Since each of the six distortions is an entirely different type of fascial deformation, proprioceptive and nociceptive information will be different, and each of the six fascial distortions feels different.

There is one person in the world who knows already which of the six distortions are present, due to exclusive information via a supreme sensory network – the patient. The challenge for the practitioner is to gain access to this exclusive information by communication and observation.

The main components of an FDM diagnosis

Non-verbal description of the complaints

Observation and classification of specific pain gestures. Patients all over the world, regardless of their age, education, or ethnic origin, display the same reproducible gestures, unconsciously displayed, when communicating their complaints.

Verbal description of the complaints

Listening, detection of keywords, classification of reproducible verbal description of the complaints.

Objective findings

Clinical examination, mobility tests, palpation.

Mechanism of injury

If available, the mechanism of injury is helpful information to determine the type of distortion.

Other diagnostic tools have yet to be implemented. As stated above, the implementation of other methods requires additional effort in terms of time and financial resources and must be justified, by either better sensitivity, specificity, inter-rater reliability, relevance, or other measurable benefits.

The Fascial Matrix 5

The fascial matrix is a three-dimensional biotensegrity framework of connective tissue. Adstrum, et al. (2017) define the fascial system as follows:

> The fascial system consists of the three-dimensional continuum of soft, collagen-containing, loose and dense fibrous connective tissues that permeate the body. It incorporates elements such as adipose tissue, adventitiae and neurovascular sheaths, aponeuroses, deep and superficial fasciae, epineurium, joint capsules, ligaments, membranes, meninges, myofascial expansions, periostea, retinacula, septa, tendons, visceral fasciae, and all the intramuscular and intermuscular connective tissues including endo-/peri-/epimysium. The fascial system interpenetrates and surrounds all organs, muscles, bones and nerve fibers, endowing the body with a functional structure, and providing an environment that enables all body systems to operate in an integrated manner.

The fascial matrix is ubiquitous and continuous throughout the body and can act not unlike a non-Newtonian fluid, shifting in response to applied forces.

Triggerbands

A triggerband is a distorted or twisted band within the fascial matrix. It is thought that triggerbands occur in banded fascia which are strong in the longitudinal direction, but weak when a perpendicular force is applied. When a perpendicular force is applied to a fascial band, the fibrils of the matrix separate, then the exposed ends of the fibrils quickly reattach to the nearest fibril, often resulting in a wrinkle or twist within the matrix (Figs. 5.1, 5.2 and 5.3).

A patient with a triggerband often experiences pain in a well-demarcated line that is described as a

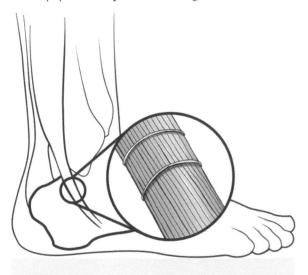

FIGURE 5.1
Banded fascia
© Kristen Janssen, used with kind permission.

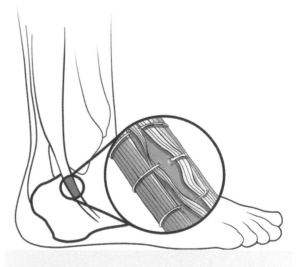

FIGURE 5.2
Triggerband
© Kristen Janssen, used with kind permission.

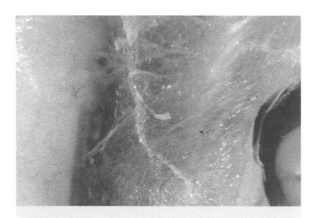

FIGURE 5.3
Triggerband found in the superficial fascia of a goat

burning, pulling, or tightness. The gesture used by the patient to describe a triggerband is a sweeping motion with the tip of one or more fingers. The fingertips will trace the exact course of the triggerband (Figs. 5.4 and 5.5).

Patients experiencing triggerbands often have reduced range of motion (ROM) in one or more planes. They may experience weakness of a limb in certain positions, while the limb remains strong in other positions. An objective loss of balance and proprioception is another common symptom.

Any place on the body where pain is demonstrated in a linear pattern with a finite start and

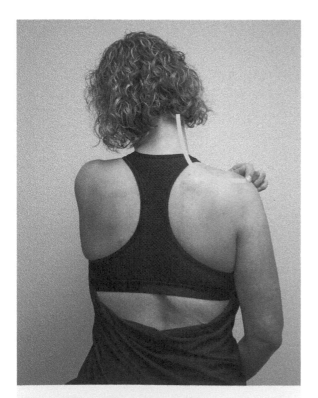

FIGURE 5.4
Shoulder–mastoid triggerband: patient gesture 1

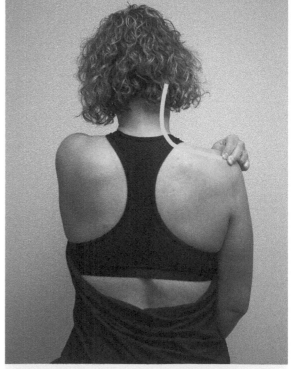

FIGURE 5.5
Shoulder–mastoid triggerband: patient gesture 2

endpoint represents a triggerband. The start and endpoints are a consistent feature, even when the patient describes them as passing through the body. Patient gestures may be limited to a short portion of the overall triggerband, either due to limitations in the patient's ROM, or because the portion indicated by the gesture is the only painful portion.

A triggerband can be palpated by the practitioner. These are frequently described as indurated and range in width from a fine line to a wide ribbon. The practitioner may elicit pain on palpation along the entire course of the triggerband, beyond the short area first identified by the patient.

Dr Typaldos described various subtypes of triggerbands. These descriptions were provided to explain the different palpatory sensations that can be felt when treating them:

Twist – the sensation appreciated when the triggerband twists during treatment (Fig. 5.6).

Wave – the sensation of the fascial tissue of the triggerband bunching up in front of the practitioner's thumb (Fig. 5.7).

Crumple – the sensation of a wave that changes depth in the fascial matrix (Fig. 5.8).

Knot – considered to be a loop in the triggerband. This knot moves along the triggerband as it is treated. Knots come in various sizes (Fig. 5.9).

Triggerband technique

Triggerband technique is a manual technique in which the practitioner uses the edge of their thumb

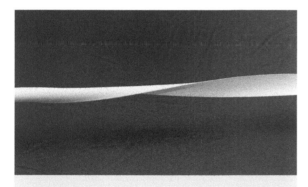

FIGURE 5.6
Twist

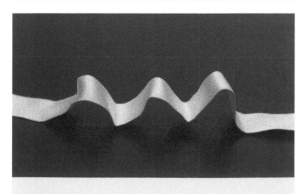

FIGURE 5.7
Wave

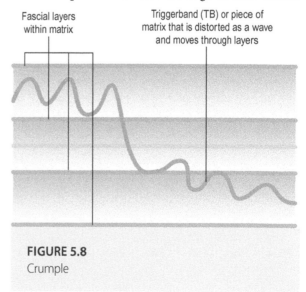

Fascial layers within matrix

Triggerband (TB) or piece of matrix that is distorted as a wave and moves through layers

FIGURE 5.8
Crumple

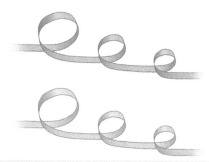

FIGURE 5.9
Knot

to apply force along the entire length of the trigger-band, untwisting the twisted fascial fibers. The force being applied to a triggerband must be directly on the skin: it should not be treated through clothes. The friction of the thumb on the skin is what allows the fibers of the fascial matrix to be separated, therefore use of lubrication between the practitioner's thumb and the patient's skin is very rarely required. The force applied by the thumb separates the twisted fascial fibers within the fascial matrix, and allows the fibrils to reattach in a more neutral or normal position.

When treating a triggerband, the practitioner should seek feedback from the patient. The patient

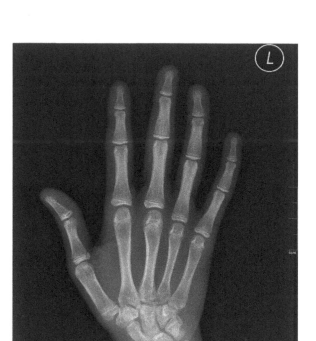

FIGURE 5.10
Hand X-ray, showing thumb
© *Nevit Dilmen, CC BY-SA 3.0, https://commons.wikimedia.org/w/index.php?curid=17361673*

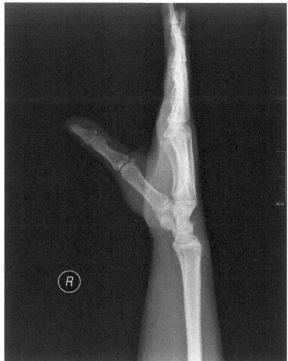

FIGURE 5.11
Thumb X-ray
© *Nevit Dilmen, CC BY-SA 3.0, https://commons.wikimedia.org/w/index.php?curid=17746494*

will describe the treatment as a cutting or burning sensation as the practitioner moves their thumb along the triggerband. If the patient feels relief, the practitioner has "fallen off" the triggerband, or the triggerband has ended. It is important to start before the origin of the triggerband and to continue the treatment all the way to the terminus. If only a portion of the triggerband is treated, the fascial matrix may remain weak, and the triggerband may easily reform.

Triggerbands are said to be acute if no fascial adhesions have formed. If adhesions have formed and are stabilizing the triggerband, it is said to be chronic. The formation of a triggerband in the fascial matrix tends to cause and recruit secondary triggerbands. The goal of every treatment is to untwist the twisted fascial fibers, reattach separated fascial fibers, and break adhesions when they are present.

When performing triggerband technique, proper thumb position is essential. The edge of the thumb is placed directly on the triggerband, positioned so that the bone located in the tip of the thumb (Figs. 5.10 and 5.11) is acting like a knife blade, cutting through the triggerband (Fig. 5.12). The practitioner pushes away from their own body and the fingers of the treating hand can be used to pull the thumb along during the treatment. The non-treating hand can adjust the tension on the skin, preventing the tissue from bunching up in front of the treating thumb. Practitioners must maintain short thumbnails to be able to treat triggerbands without leaving nail marks on the patient.

Depth and speed are vital aspects of triggerband technique. If the practitioner thinks of their thumb as a farmer's plow (Fig. 5.13), they can adjust the angle and depth to obtain the proper depth of treatment (Fig. 5.14). Using the proper depth improves the effectiveness of the treatment, minimizes the force required, and often can make the treatment much more tolerable for the patient. A triggerband can easily be treated too fast: the practitioner's thumb then slides across the skin, and there is not adequate friction to separate the underlying fascial fibers. If treatment is unsuccessful, slow the treatment down, press deeper into the tissue, and consider changing the direction of treatment. The correct speed of triggerband treatment is the speed at which the tissue can be felt changing under the treating thumb.

With practice and constant feedback from patients, practitioners gain ever-improving palpatory

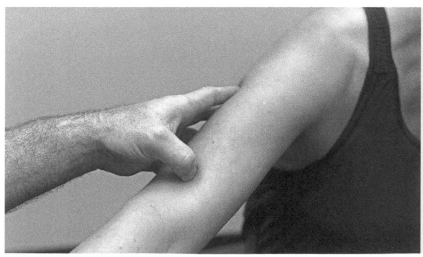

FIGURE 5.12
Triggerband technique thumb placement

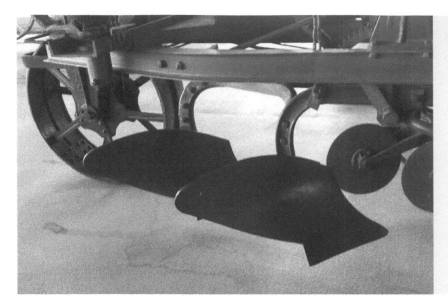

FIGURE 5.13
An antique two-furrow plow

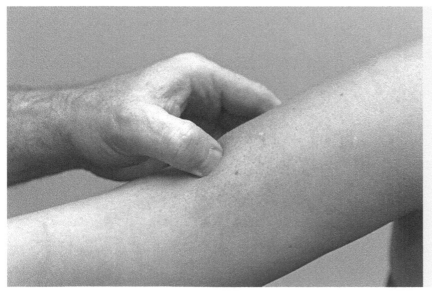

FIGURE 5.14
Angling the thumb like a
plow blade

skills and learn to feel the location and depth of the triggerbands as they treat them. When learning how to treat a triggerband, the practitioner must trust that the exact location provided by the patient is where it is located. The location is confirmed by patient feedback regarding the pain that is experienced. If the pain of the treatment disappears, the triggerband is either finished or has been lost along the course of the treatment.

The direction of triggerband treatment can also make a difference in the outcome of triggerband technique. Often, treatment is in the direction that the patient first demonstrates the triggerband, but if the initial pass is not successful, reversing the direction of treatment may be helpful. The practitioner can start and stop during treatment, to work around clothing or to switch thumbs, as long as they note the triggerband pathway, make necessary adjustments, and take a step back along the triggerband course before resuming treatment.

Triggerbands can have a variety of clinical progressions. They can heal slowly; they may remain acute regardless of duration if adhesions do not form; or they may form adhesions and become chronic in a relatively short time. Alternatively, they can be repaired immediately with triggerband technique.

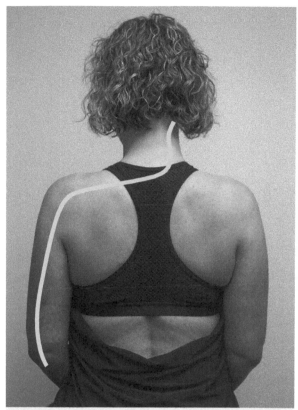

FIGURE 5.16
Posterior shoulder triggerband

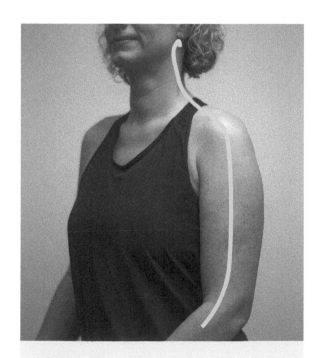

FIGURE 5.15
Anterior shoulder triggerband

Every FDM practitioner should be aware of common triggerband pathways and their general location. The patient is always the expert, and they will guide the practitioner to the location of their specific triggerband either with their body language or by the reaction to triggerband treatment. Common pathways are the anterior shoulder triggerband (Fig. 5.15), posterior shoulder triggerband (Fig. 5.16), shoulder–mastoid triggerband (Fig. 5.17), lumbar triggerband (Fig. 5.18), posterior thigh triggerband (Fig. 5.19), lateral thigh triggerband (Fig. 5.20) and lateral ankle triggerband (Fig. 5.21).

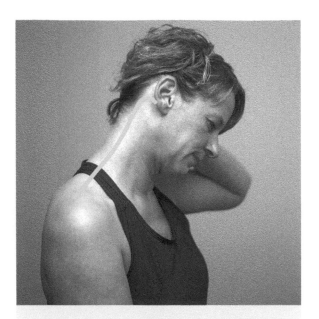

FIGURE 5.17
Shoulder–mastoid triggerband

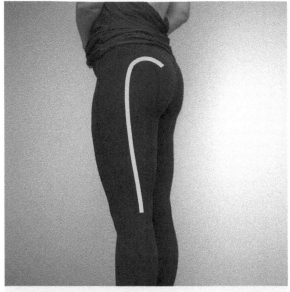

FIGURE 5.19
Posterior thigh triggerband

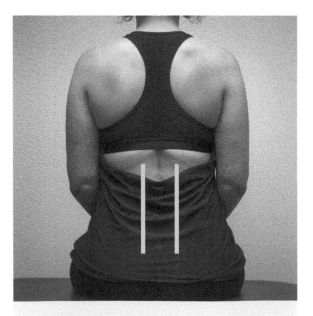

FIGURE 5.18
Lumbar triggerband

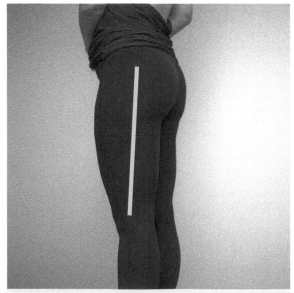

FIGURE 5.20
Lateral thigh triggerband

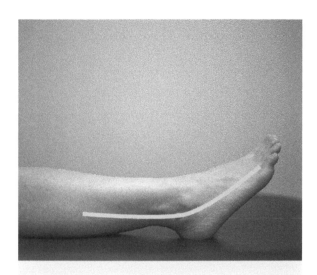

FIGURE 5.21
Lateral ankle triggerband

Triggerband thumb

The force required to treat a triggerband can distort the fascia in the practitioner's thumb, causing a condition called "triggerband thumb" (see also p. 166). Distortions commonly found in cases of triggerband thumb include folding distortions (FDs) of the thumb joints and triggerbands along the thumb.

Triggerbands

- Body language: sweeping or drawing a line with the tips of the fingers along the exact route of the triggerband

- Verbal descriptors: "pulling, burning, tightness"

- Treatment:

  - Triggerband technique: iron out the twisted fascial band with the edge of the thumbtip.

  - Be sure to treat the entire pathway: partial treatment may allow the triggerband to reform.

Herniated triggerpoints (HTPs)

The second distortion discovered by Dr Typaldos was the herniated triggerpoint (HTP), thought to be the abnormal protrusion of tissue through the smooth fascial plane. HTPs can form anywhere on the body in the fascial matrix. Initially, they were thought to occur randomly throughout the body; however, it is now hypothesized that the passage of neurovascular bundles through the fascial matrix creates an inherent weakness in the matrix, providing an avenue for tissue to herniate or protrude within it (Fig. 5.22). The protruding tissue is often fascial tissue.

When a patient has an HTP, they will often press into a painful spot in soft tissue with multiple fingers, a thumb, or a knuckle (see Figs. 5.23 and 5.24). Patients will sometimes speak of the relief they feel when pressure is applied to the distinctly painful spot. They may use their own hands, a tool or asked others to apply pressure to the painful areas. The patient intuitively knows that reducing the herniated tissue

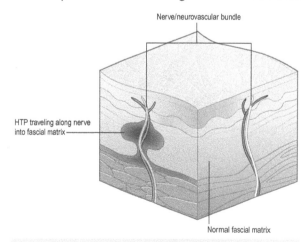

FIGURE 5.22
Neurovascular bundles traveling through the fascial matrix

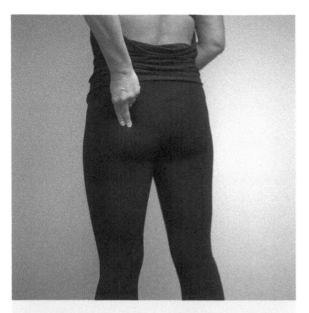

FIGURE 5.23
Two fingers pressing into a painful spot, indicating presence and location of a herniated trigger point (HTP)

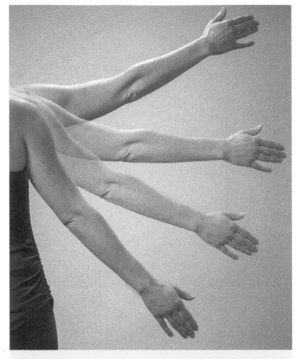

FIGURE 5.25
"Racheting" motion secondary to a herniated trigger point (HTP)

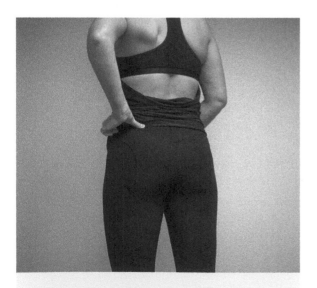

FIGURE 5.24
Thumb pressing into a painful spot, indicating presence and location of a herniated trigger point (HTP)

back below the fascial plane will provide relief. When experiencing an HTP, a patient may complain of pinching, catching, or a local dull ache, and they may cause a decreased ROM of contiguous joints. HTPs may be detectable upon palpation by the patient and provider or appreciated as a painful "knots" in the soft tissue. HTPs may disrupt the fluid movement of a joint or extremity. This disrupted movement is described as stepping or ratcheting (Fig. 5.25). Fluid movement in the affected joint may be partially restored when pressure is applied to the HTP.

HTP treatment

Treatment of an HTP involves the practitioner using their thumb to reduce the herniated tissue back below the tissue plane that it has protruded into (Fig. 5.26). The goal of every HTP treatment is the complete reduction of the herniated tissue and the subsequent closure of the hole in the plane through which the tissue protruded.

HTPs are best located by observing the patient's gesture and then palpating the area described. The practitioner should work to appreciate the subtle soft tissue changes near the area of the complaint through superficial palpation. Once the approximate location of the HTP is determined, firmer palpation can be applied, and patient input should be sought to verify precisely where the HTP is located. While applying pressure, it is important to take note of the angle or vector that causes the patient the most tenderness as this angle is often the angle at which force must be applied to reduce the HTP.

The force applied when reducing an HTP should begin with a gradual increase of pressure until tension in the tissue is maximized. The thumb is then thrust through the fascial plane, reducing the protruding tissue below the plane. Often a "squish" of the tissues is appreciated when the HTP is reduced.

When reducing an HTP, it is crucial to leave no portion of the HTP stuck in the fascial plane. Failure to completely reduce the HTP can lead to sharp or pinching pain that may be worse than the patient's initial complaint. If the HTP is partially reduced and the patient complains of increased pain, the provider should palpate the firm area of protruding tissue and force it below the fascial plane (Fig. 5.27). The fascial plane through which the protruding tissue will be reduced can be neither too taut nor too loose. If the tissue plane is too taut, the herniated tissue cannot be pressed through the plane; if it is too loose, there will be no resistance, or insufficient resistance, to the pressure of the practitioner's thumb. The very tip of the thumb should be utilized to force the protruding tissue through the fascial plane. If the flat of the

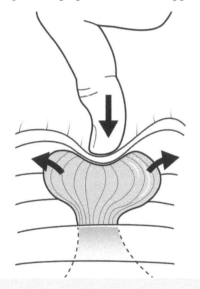

FIGURE 5.26
Reduction of a herniated triggerpoint (HTP)
© *Kristen Janssen, used with kind permission.*

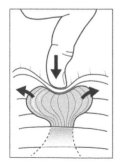
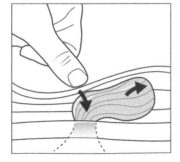
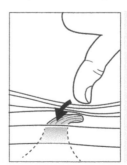

FIGURE 5.27
Ensuring the complete reduction of a herniated triggerpoint (HTP)
© *Kristen Janssen, used with kind permission.*

thumb is used, or anything larger than the tip of the thumb (such as an elbow or knuckle), the probability of successful reduction is dramatically reduced.

An appropriate sequence of treatment for an HTP would include:

- observing the patient's gesture indicating an HTP
- palpation of the HTP
- verification of the most tender area
- reduction of the protruding tissue below the fascial plane
- palpation for firm residual edges of protruding through the fascial plane
- tucking any remaining tissue edges below the fascial plane.

Once the HTP is reduced, the tension of the fascial matrix works to close the opening through which tissue has herniated. This closure can take some time – some references suggest 90 minutes – and if the body is delayed in closing this tissue, then recurrence of the HTP is possible. Hydration appears to play a significant role in the timely and efficient closure of the matrix.

HTPs may occur suddenly, such as those formed by a traumatic event. They can also develop slowly and insidiously, when sleeping or in a prolonged sedentary position. It is thought that once the tissue of the HTP has herniated, physiologic movement is insufficient to reduce the HTP without external intervention, and so HTPs are considered permanent until reduced. This characteristic of HTPs makes them a commonly found distortion in patients with long-standing pain.

There are two subtypes of HTPs: banded and non-banded HTPs. Non-banded HTPs are formed when a small opening in the fascial matrix has allowed the passage of material through the fascial plane. The tissue that has protruded through the plane is larger in diameter than the opening through which it came. This enlargement makes the spontaneous reduction of the protruded tissue unlikely. The image of a mushroom with a large top and narrow base can be used to visualize the non-banded HTP.

Banded HTPs are HTPs associated with trigger-bands as it is the triggerband in the tissue plane of the fascial matrix that prevents the reduction of the protruding tissue. Treatment of the triggerband may be required to facilitate reduction of the HTP and may also be required for complete closure of the involved fascial plane following the reduction of the HTP.

Fascial rent

When treating an HTP, initial reduction is often followed by quick palpation for firm residual edges that need to be tucked below the fascial plane. When this firm edge continues in a linear path, the concept of the HTP resembling a mushroom is no longer accurate, and instead there appears to be a linear opening, or rent, in the tissue plane that has allowed a protrusion of tissue along this opening (see Chapter 8, Fig. 8.11.) This was previously mistakenly referred to as the "banding" of an HTP, leading to confusion between the subtypes of non-banded and banded HTPs, but when a larger portion of the tissue plane appears to have opened accompanied by a linear protrusion of tissue, this is now referred to as a **fascial rent**. Treatment of this type of HTP is the same as for other types: the tender spot identified by the patient is palpated, and then the tip of the thumb is used to reduce the herniated tissue below the affected fascial plane along the entire length of the protruding tissue.

Common HTPs include the supraclavicular HTP (SCHTP) (Fig. 5.28), deltoid HTP (Fig. 5.29), scapulothoracic HTP (Fig. 5.30), bullseye HTP (Fig. 5.31), and flank HTP (Fig. 5.32). It is important to recall

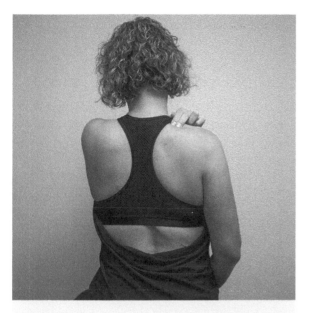

FIGURE 5.28
Supraclavicular herniated trigger point (HTP)

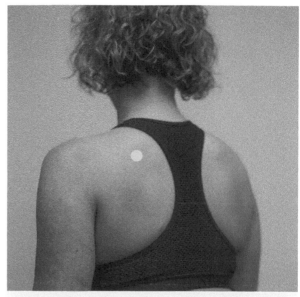

FIGURE 5.30
Scapulothoracic herniated trigger point (HTP)

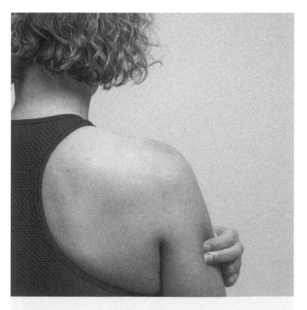

FIGURE 5.29
Deltoid herniated trigger point (HTP)

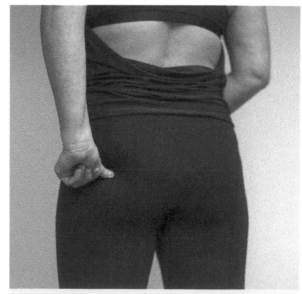

FIGURE 5.31
Bullseye herniated trigger point (HTP)

that HTPs occur wherever the patient identifies them on the body, including the extremities, head, trunk, and abdomen.

Herniated triggerpoints (HTPs)

- Body language: pressing into a soft tissue area with multiple fingers, a thumb, or a knuckle

- Verbal descriptors: aching, tightness

- Treatment:

    - Reduction of herniated tissue below fascial plane with tip of thumb.

    - An increase in pain, or sensation of sharp, pinching pain at the reduction site should prompt the practitioner to search for and reduce any remaining tails of fascia.

Continuum distortions (CDs)

The third distortion identified by Dr Typaldos was the continuum distortion (CD). A patient identifies the CD as a single spot of pain on a bone or between tissue types, gesturing with a single finger pressing onto the painful spot (Fig. 5.33).

It is important to understand that every fascia–bone connection represents a transition zone in which the soft tissue matrix of the fascia blends into the bone. This transition zone is constantly shifting between rigid and flexible states (Fig. 5.34) and the transition between flexible and rigid is the result of a calcium flux into or out of the transition zone, known as a continuum. Every bone and fascia intersection is therefore a continuum and has the potential to be distorted.

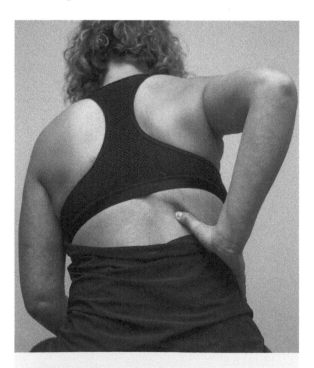

FIGURE 5.32
Flank herniated trigger point (HTP)

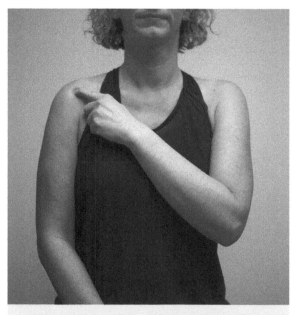

FIGURE 5.33
A single finger pressing onto a painful spot, indicating presence and location of a continuum distortion (CD)

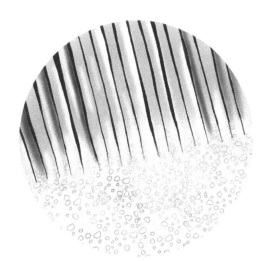

FIGURE 5.34
The transition zone
© *Kristen Janssen, used with kind permission.*

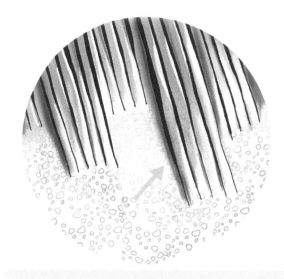

FIGURE 5.36
Inverted continuum distortion (CD)
© *Kristen Janssen, used with kind permission.*

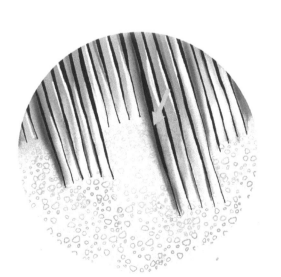

FIGURE 5.35
Everted continuum distortion (CD)
© *Kristen Janssen, used with kind permission.*

The transition zone between bone and fascia is thought to regulate tissue stiffness and flexibility of the intersection in response to loads applied to the fascial matrix in that region. If calcium moves into the transition zone (continuum), then the intersection becomes more rigid. If calcium is absorbed back into the bone, the transition zone becomes more flexible. This continuum will become distorted when the transition zone is stuck and unable to shift between the rigid and flexible state. A CD is defined as the alteration of the transition zone between the bone and the fascial covering of ligament or tendon that prevents the transition zone from shifting normally.

If calcium is stuck in the transition zone, this is called an **everted continuum distortion** (everted CD) (Fig. 5.35). Calcium stuck in the transition zone is appreciated as a tender calcific spot on the bone. These tender spicules of bone vary in size, but are often 3–5mm. If calcium is stuck in the bone and unable to move out to the transition zone, this is termed an **inverted continuum distortion** (inverted CD) (Fig. 5.36). Inverted CDs feel like a divot in the bone and are often compared to the hole found in a belt.

CDs are tender to palpation and are thought to occur in the banded fascia of the fascial matrix. Essentially, the CD occurs where banded fascia transitions to the bone.

CD treatment

The physical gesture a patient will use to demonstrate a CD is a single finger identifying a single spot of pain on the bone. Careful observation of the gesture can assist in the reduction of the CD, as the gesture will often include the vector that should be replicated when treating, often the most painful angle or vector. When treating a CD with continuum technique, the very tip of the practitioner's thumb palpates the area identified by the

patient (Fig. 5.37). After the practitioner locates the most tender area of the fascia–bone connection, treatment may commence. Treatment is intense and should be brief, lasting only seconds. When the proper direction of force is achieved, pressure on the transition zone is increased until a sudden shift or change in the transition zone is appreciated. When this happens, the practitioner should immediately stop the treatment and re-assess. It is easy to miss the subtle sensation of the shifting transition zone, but the ability to appreciate the shift should improve as the palpatory abilities of the provider's thumb improves. CD treatments are an "all or none" treatment (Typaldos, 1995). Either the transition zone has shifted, or it has not: there is no partial treatment of a CD. As the practitioner gains experience, learning to sense the shift in the continuum will help reduce the amount of unnecessary pain associated with treatment. By using only the necessary force and duration when treating CDs, the provider will also prevent fatigue in their thumb.

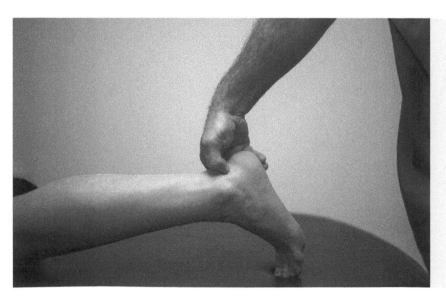

FIGURE 5.37
Thumb placement for continuum technique

Once a CD is treated, and the patient is reassessed for pain, they may identify other CDs that are very close to the initially identified distortion. These clusters of CDs are thought to occur when a portion of the banded fascia pulls on the zone of transition between bone and ligament in the affected area. The initial CD is the most painful spot and therefore the one that the patient initially identifies. As the most painful area is treated, the patient can identify other areas of pain. Working through multiple CDs in an area of pain is not unusual.

CDs appear to be related to a sudden change in the demands placed on the fascia–bone transition zone. For example, in the case of a sprain-type injury, the transition zone is stressed before the body can react or adjust calcium distribution to alter tissue tension in the transition zone. CDs are commonly found in injuries with a sprain-type mechanism or any injury of a sudden nature.

In the FDM, some types of fractures are thought to be the extension of a CD into the bone. In fractures, the bone–ligament transition zone has been stressed to the point that the bony matrix is damaged, and the site of the bony disruption will commonly have painful tender spots that represent the CDs. These spots can be addressed with continuum technique if within the scope of the provider's practice, allowing for reduction of pain associated with the fracture.

Restriction of ROM in one plane is a common physical finding associated with CDs. An everted CD can be palpated and appreciated as a small, calcific tender area on the periosteum of the bone while an inverted CD is often palpated and appreciated as a small indent in the periosteum at the exact spot identified by the patient, and is very painful when pressure is applied. Continuum technique can be used for both inverted and everted CDs. Direct pressure with the bony portion of the tip of the thumb directly onto the most tender bony area of the CD is applied until the continuum shifts. In the case of the inverted CDs, if direct continuum technique is not effective, then a traction thrust technique can be utilized to pull the calcium from the bone, not unlike pulling dents out of a car body. With inverted CDs, proper positioning can take up the slack in the soft tissue, enabling the banded fascia to pull the calcium out of the inverted CD when a thrust mobilization is applied.

The goal of every CD treatment is to restore the normal physiologic ability of the continuum to shift freely between the states of the transition zone, i.e. the fascial state and the bony state. There is no partial success when treating CDs. The natural progression of CDs is variable: they may heal on their own or come and go with activity.

Both CDs and triggerbands occur in banded fascia and CDs may be associated with triggerbands. One way to visualize the CD–triggerband relationship is to think of a cable connecting to a rigid spot. The cable may have a twist (triggerband), and the anchor point may have a disruption (CD).

While CDs are most commonly believed to occur between fascia and bone, Dr Typaldos suggested that the transition zone between any tissue type had a continuum and therefore could be the site of CD formation.

CDs are found wherever the patient shows them. Common CDs include occipital CD (Fig. 5.38), anterior ankle CD (Fig. 5.39), sacral CD (Fig. 5.40), calcaneal CD (Fig. 5.41) and lateral epicondyle CD (Fig. 5.42).

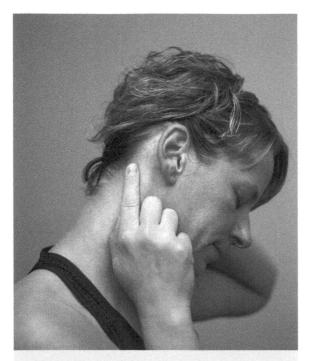

FIGURE 5.38
Occipital continuum distortion (CD)

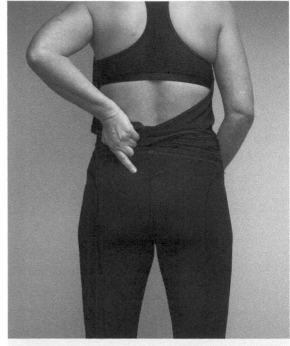

FIGURE 5.40
Sacral continuum distortion (CD)

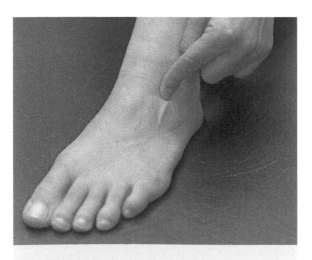

FIGURE 5.39
Anterior ankle continuum distortion (CD)

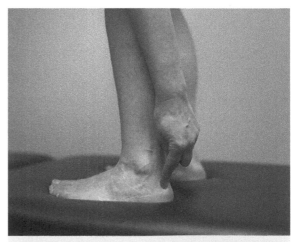

FIGURE 5.41
Calcaneal continuum distortion (CD)

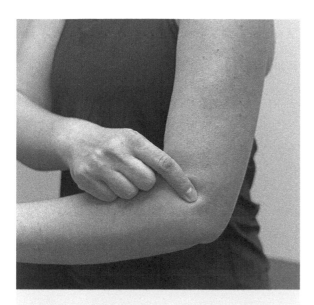

FIGURE 5.42
Lateral epicondyle continuum distortion (CD)

Folding distortions (FDs)

Folding distortions (FDs) are a three-dimensional alteration of the fascial plane. The fascial matrix can compress and expand to absorb and dissipate forces. When forces applied to the matrix cause the fascial network to expand, this is called unfolding. Conversely, when a compressive force deforms the matrix, it is called refolding. Unfolding and refolding of the fascial matrix can be visualized as a spring-like shock absorber.

Folding fascia functions throughout the body, protecting the body from injury. It is commonly seen in the spine, but is also present between every muscle, all joints, and between the organs.

FD treatment

It is paramount to remember that the treatment of FDs should be painless. If the patient expresses pain while being treated for a FD, either one of the painful distortions remains in the matrix, or the treatment is being performed in the direction opposite to that required to restore function of the matrix.

The physical gesture associated with an FD is that of the patient holding or cupping the area that is distorted with their hand (Fig. 5.43). Patients will often experience a deep ache inside the body, but will be unable to pinpoint or precisely locate the pain. The phrase "it is somewhere in there" is commonly used to help identify the origin of their pain. Patients may experience significant pain in the area without major loss of ROM. They may note that the pain changes with the weather, and may have the perception that the joint or area involved feels unstable, despite the area remaining structurally stable on physical examination. These injuries can last a long time, and patients will often feel like they have "always" had the pain.

The unfolding and refolding mechanism is considered to be distorted when the matrix is stuck in one of these two states and unable to move to the other state.

Continuum distortions (CDs)

- Body language: pointing with a single finger to a bony spot

- Verbal descriptors: Patient will identify a single, discrete point of pain

- Objective finding: restricted ROM in one plane

- Treatment:

  - Reduction of shifted continuum material by application of pressure from the tip of the practitioner's thumb.

  - Pay attention to the angle of the patient's finger when they are showing where the CD is: this angle is often the angle needed for reduction of the CD.

Treating a refolding distortion (rFD)

If a compressive force is applied to the fascial matrix, accompanied by another force that distorts the matrix (torque), the matrix can become stuck in compression, or refolded (Fig. 5.44). An example of this type of injury might be a fall on an outstretched arm. The mechanism of injury is a compression and a twist, which then causes the matrix to be stuck in compression. These injuries are called refolding distortions (rFDs). While all folding injuries are recognized by the holding or cupping of an area, rFDs may present with the additional gesture of a line being drawn across the joint (Fig. 5.45).

Treatment of a refolding is performed by repeating the mechanism of injury. A compression injury

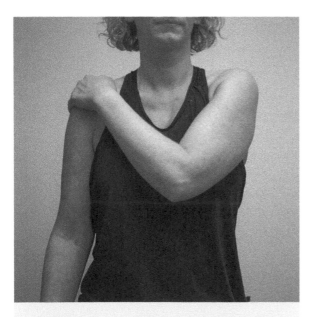

FIGURE 5.43
Holding/cupping a painful area, indicating presence and location of a folding distortion (FD)

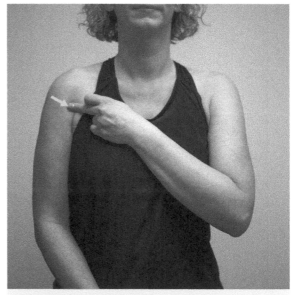

FIGURE 5.45
Drawing a line across the affected area, indicating presence and location of folding distortion (FD)

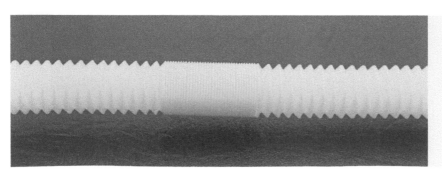

FIGURE 5.44
Simulation of an area of folding fascia stuck in a folded state

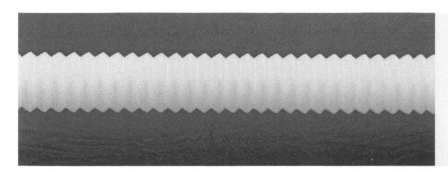

FIGURE 5.46
Simulation of an area of folding fascia stuck in an unfolded state

requires compression to be treated. Many practitioners mistakenly attempt to treat folding injuries by forcing the matrix into the state that it is unable to transition towards, essentially unfolding a refolding injury. This is not correct, and could (and often does) cause pain. Refolding injuries need to be refolded. The direction and force of the refolding is the same as that which caused the initial injury.

Treatment of folding injuries should be painless. The tissue should be refolded in the direction that is painless and feels correct to the patient.

Treating an unfolding distortion (uFD)

When the fascial matrix overexpands in conjunction with a torsional force resulting in the matrix being stuck in an unfolded state, the matrix is said to have an unfolding distortion (uFD) (Fig. 5.46). For example, consider a person walking a dog on a leash. If the dog suddenly pulls on the leash, the person's shoulder can be pulled in an unusual or unanticipated direction, leading to a uFD. Unfolding injuries need to be treated by unfolding them, removing the impediment, and allowing the fascial matrix to return to the normal transition between refolding and unfolding.

uFDs feel worse with compression and improve with traction. uFDs are often associated with edema at the site of the distortion, thought to be the body's

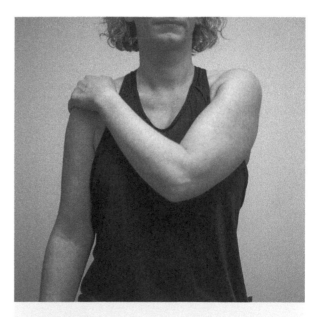

FIGURE 5.47
Shoulder folding distortion (FD)

own attempt at treating the uFD. When fluid is pushed into a joint, the tissue unfolds, and when the fluid is reabsorbed, the tissue is able to refold.

Examples of frequent FD gestures include shoulder FD (Fig. 5.47), knee FD (Fig. 5.48), lumbar FD (Fig. 5.49), intermuscular septal FD of upper arm (Fig. 5.50), interosseous membrane FD of forearm (Fig. 5.51), jaw FD (Fig. 5.52), and FD headache (Fig. 5.53).

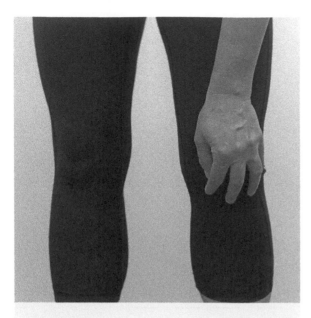

FIGURE 5.48
Knee folding distortion (FD)

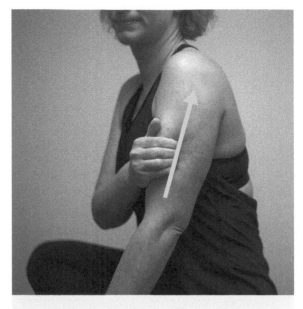

FIGURE 5.50
Intermuscular septal folding distortion (FD) in upper arm

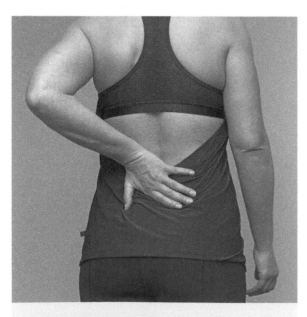

FIGURE 5.49
Lumbar folding distortion (FD)

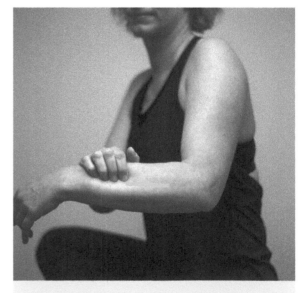

FIGURE 5.51
Interosseous membrane folding distortion (FD) of forearm

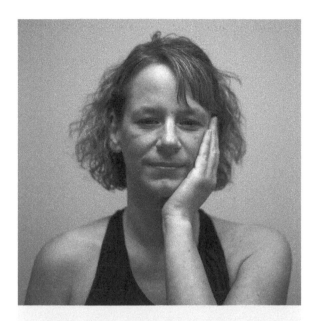

FIGURE 5.52
Jaw folding distortion (FD)

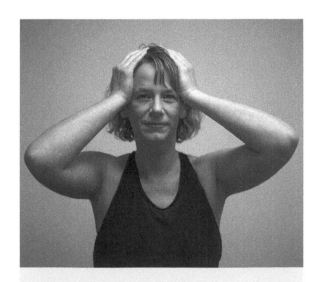

FIGURE 5.53
Folding distortion (FD) headache

Folding distortions (FDs)

- Body language: holding or cupping the affected area with the hand

- Verbal descriptors: pain deep in the affected body part without ability to articulate exactly where

- Treatment:

  - Should be painless. Patient feedback is paramount to success.

  - Recreates the mechanism of injury.

Cylinder distortions (CyDs)

Cylinder distortions (CyDs) are thought to occur in the circular or coiled fascia. It is hypothesized that the circular fascia is the most superficial fascia, found just below the skin. These circular coils of the fascial matrix can be visualized as a spring or coil that encircles the body, sliding below the skin (Fig. 5.54). The coils must be able to slide and move uninhibited, or the body interprets the restriction of these fascial coils as pain. When fascial coils are constricted or inhibited, they can be thought of as "kinked" (Fig. 5.55) and the practitioner's job is to unkink the coils of circular fascia and restore fluid movement.

The etiology behind the formation of CyDs is not always readily identified; however, restriction of the skin movement on the underlying circular fascia, as seen with splints, casts, wraps, bandages, and tight or compressive garments, may lead to the tangling of these coils.

A patient who is experiencing a CyD may gesture with the palm of their hand or pads of their fingers while squeezing, sweeping, wringing, or wiping

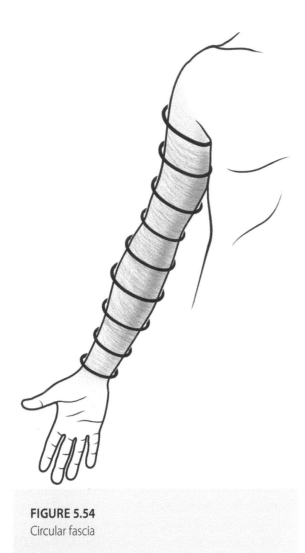

FIGURE 5.54
Circular fascia

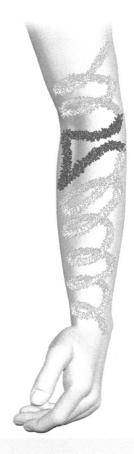

FIGURE 5.55
"Kinked" coils of circular fascia
Based on an original drawing by Brianna Regan Davis, used with kind permission

the area of pain. The gesture may appear as though they are trying to remove water from their skin or to remove an invisible garment such as a glove or sock (Fig. 5.56). Patients with a CyD may gesture without contacting their body, instead passing their hands over the affected area (Fig. 5.57). Another gesture associated with the CyD is the drawing of a circle on the skin. This circular shape could be related to an underlying distortion (such as an HTP) causing a superficial disruption of the coiled fascia.

Gesturing with a c-shaped hand may also indicate a CyDis present.

Patients experiencing CyDs will often describe bizarre pain. Patients may find it difficult to adequately explain the pain, or report that the pain jumps from one area to another, is felt deep in the body, and is of inexplicable intensity. At times they will describe the sensation of the region being swollen even though there is no evidence of actual swelling. Patients may experience paresthesias, tingling, tremors, fasciculation, or cramping. These types of pain described may not follow traditional anatomical distribution, causing medical providers to be skeptical. When a patient presents with any

bizarre or unusual symptoms, consideration should be given to the presence of a CyD.

CyDs may cause pain in active motion but be relatively pain-free in passive motion. The pain experienced may appear out of proportion to physical findings. In general, a CyD is not thought to be something a provider can palpate; however, the coils of fascia can occasionally bunch up to the extent that there is a palpable coil under the skin surface. Dr Typaldos spoke of using a medium bristle pet comb to comb or pull out the tangles of the fascia. This comb technique can often highlight these ridges of bunched up fascia as the comb is dragged across the skin surface.

CyD treatment

The goal of CyD treatment is to untangle the tangled coils of fascial and restore the normal movement of the circular fascia. Often the skin can be raised or pulled away from the underlying fascia, allowing the kinked coils to move back to their neutral distribution. Cupping with movement

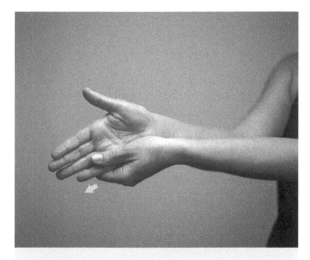

FIGURE 5.56
Wiping/squeezing the area of pain, indicating presence and location of a cylinder distortion (CyD)

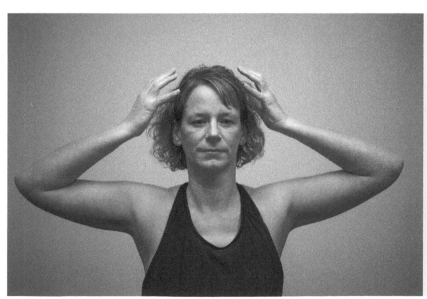

FIGURE 5.57
Passing hands over the area of pain without contact, indicating presence and location of a cylinder distortion (CyD)

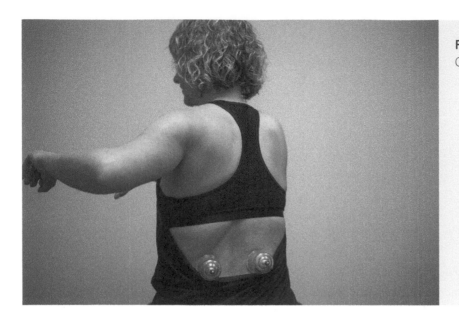

FIGURE 5.58
Cupping with movement

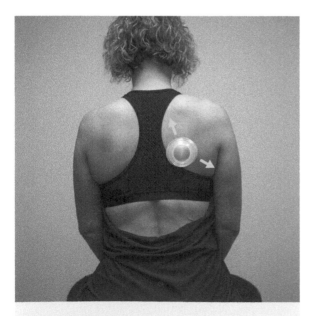

FIGURE 5.59
Cupping with sliding

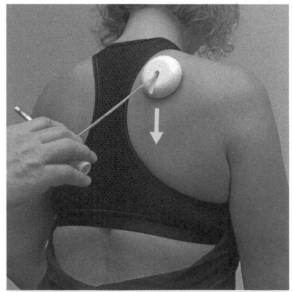

FIGURE 5.60
Vacuum extractor cupping with sliding

(Fig. 5.58), cupping with sliding (Fig. 5.59), the use of the vacuum extractor (Fig. 5.60), tiger claw (Fig. 5.61), and plunger techniques (Fig. 5.62) pull the skin away from the underlying fascial coils. While the skin is pulled away, the patient may provide movement to further free up the coils. Additionally, manual treatments such as the squeegee (Fig. 5.63), snake bite, skin rolling (Fig. 5.64), and double-thumb techniques (Fig. 5.65) can be employed to move the fascial coils through direct friction applied to the skin.

While the goal of every cylinder technique is to untangle the kinked fascial coils, the practitioner must proceed with caution, as overtreatment of CyD can make matters worse. CyDs are thought to be the only distortion that can be caused by the practitioner with treatment. The natural progression of the CyD can be just as bizarre as its presentation as cylinders often behave unpredictably.

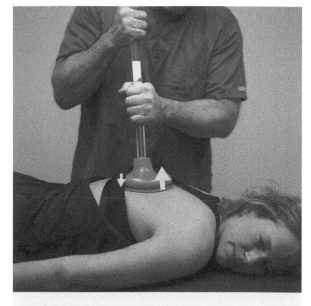

FIGURE 5.62
Plunger technique

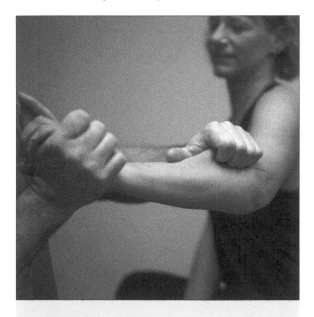

FIGURE 5.61
Tiger claw technique

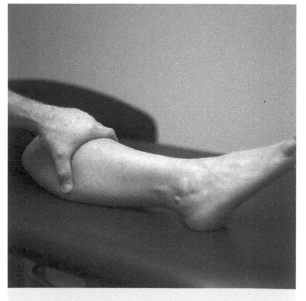

FIGURE 5.63
Squeegee technique

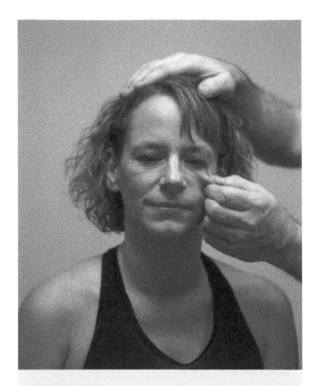

FIGURE 5.64
Skin rolling technique

Cylinder distortions (CyDs)

- Body language:

    - Sweeping, wringing, or wiping affected area with palm or pads of fingers

    - The gesturing hand may not contact the affected area

- Verbal descriptors:

    - Bizarre, difficult to explain pain

    - May jump from one area of body to another

    - May report pain of unusual intensity

- Treatment: separate the tangled coils of cylindrical fascia via manual techniques or with clips, cups, plungers, and other assistive devices.

Tectonic fixations (TFs)

A tectonic fixation (TF) is defined as the inability of the fascial surfaces to glide. TFs are thought to occur in the smooth fascia of the fascial matrix. Smooth

FIGURE 5.65
Double-thumb technique

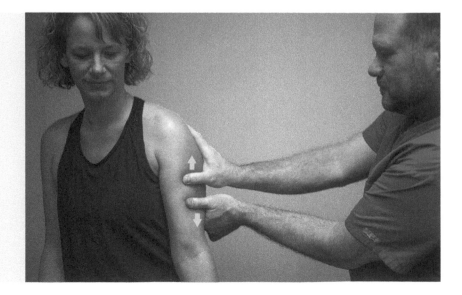

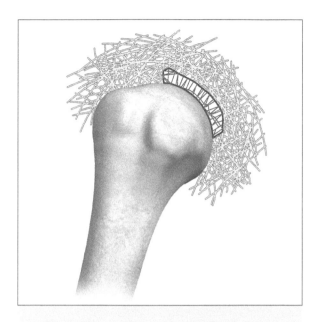

FIGURE 5.66
Tectonic fixation (TF)
Based on an original drawing by Brianna Regan Davis, used with kind permission.

fascia is visualized as layers of fascia that slide and glide on each other when a force is applied to the fascial matrix. A small amount of fluid between each layer allows the layers of tissue to slide on each other. When normal mobility is disrupted (for instance, in the presence of external immobilization, one of the other five fascial distortions, or if something decreases the amount of fluid between the layers) then the layers of fascia can become "stuck" together. When this happens, the fascial matrix has a significantly decreased ROM (Fig. 5.66).

There is no specific gesture for TF. Patients often feel that some part of their body needs to "pop" or crack when they have a TF, and may be observed doing so. They often feel like there is decreased fluid in the joint, that the joint or tissue is dry, or that it feels "low on oil."

TFs manifest as reduced ROM in the affected area and, in contrast to the other established fascial distortions, a TF is painless. Investigation of complaints of pain in a tectonically-fixed area will often reveal the presence of one of the other (painful) distortions. The patient will also often have a history of trauma or some other painful condition that limited motion in the area that now has the TF. They may have been immobilized as part of a medical intervention, or they may have self-immobilized by reducing their ROM to avoid pain.

Physical examination of a TF reveals a loss of passive ROM. There is often a rigid, bony end-feel when a tectonically-fixed joint is moved through its ROM. TFs are not painful to palpate, and there is no pain on pressure unless a painful distortion is present.

TF treatment

The goal of TF treatment is to increase the fluid between the fascial layers, pumping fluid through the fixed tissue and then forcing those fascial layers to slide. This can be assisted by heating the fixed tissue. Once the area is heated, a slow tectonic pump of the area is performed to help drive fluid between the fascial layers by moving the tissue in the matrix. The slow tectonic pump can be performed for many minutes. Some techniques utilized to treat FDs can also be used to address tectonic fascial surfaces; for example, the frog-leg technique can be used as part of the tectonic pump treatment of the shoulder. Many high-velocity, low-amplitude (HVLA) techniques are viewed as primarily treating TFs. The plunger technique may also be used to mobilize larger sections of tissue, and other medical treatments, such as intraarticular joint injection and hydrodissection, can be viewed within the FDM as working on tectonically-fixed tissue. Manipulation under general anesthesia (MUGA) is an extreme form of TF treatment, and joint replacement is the ultimate tectonic treatment, as it removes the tectonically-fixed tissue entirely.

The goal of every TF treatment is to restore the physiologic ability of the fascial surfaces to glide. Due to the tenacious nature of the TF, frequent and repeated treatment is often required. Treatment twice a week for 6 or more weeks is recommended and cups, plungers, and manual pumping techniques can be used to mobilize tissue and pull the fascial layers apart.

Frozen joints and scars can be envisioned as TFs. A scar is often observed as having a tectonic component. Evaluating scars through the lens of the FDM can introduce different thought processes when treating scars and the symptoms associated with them.

TFs are thought to begin slowly due to the presence of other painful distortions. Patients avoid moving the affected body part with these painful distortions, or only move within a pain-free ROM, allowing fascial surfaces to stick together. Scarring and reduction in ROM are not the only cause of TFs, however. Any medical condition that causes the tissue to become sticky or reduces hydration in the fascial layers can lead to a TF; for example, radiation treatments can often cause TF in the associated tissues.

Tectonic fixations (TFs)

- Body language:
    - No specific gesture
    - Attempts at self-mobilization may be observed or described
- Verbal descriptors:
    - Affected area feels "stuck, stiff, or needs to pop"
- Treatment:
    - Restore the gliding quality of the affected tissue
    - The only distortion in which application of heat may assist with treatment
    - Other painful distortions may be present and requiring treatment before addressing the TF

The following chapters present a number of complaints commonly encountered in clinical practice. Evaluating and treating these complaints through the lens of the Fascial Distortion Model (FDM) can lead to improved patient outcomes. It is worth noting that although the list of included complaints and treatments is far from exhaustive, once the practitioner uses and understands FDM, complaints not addressed in this text can easily be evaluated and treated in the model. As always, the practitioner must exercise good clinical judgement, perform appropriate physical examinations, and work within their scope of practice.

The following chapters have been divided by commonly accepted divisions in body region. This is an artifact of the codification and teaching process and should in no way be construed to indicate that a fascial distortion must be limited to the region as it is described here. It has been established that the body's fascial network is contiguous and ubiquitous; therefore fascial distortions can and do extend across multiple body regions. To use a common truism of clinical medicine, "the patient didn't read the book." The patient will guide the practitioner.

Head

Many complaints of pain involve the head. Evaluating and treating these complaints within the FDM can guide diagnosis and bring rapid relief to the patient. While there are several specific conditions with well-accepted pathologic mechanisms, these explanations do not preclude the use of, and in many cases they are quite compatible with, FDM treatment.

All six of the distortions can present in the head region. Working with the definitions of the distortions, following the patient's gestures, and listening to their verbal description will guide the practitioner and lead to pain reduction and improved function.

Headache

Headache is a common complaint with a myriad of possible causes. The FDM practitioner views these conditions as one or more of the distortions first, only moving down the list of possible differential diagnoses if treatment of the distortions presented is unsuccessful or if some signs or symptoms are concerning enough and warrant investigation in a more traditional medical thought process.

Triggerband headaches

Patients with this type of headache will often describe precise lines of pain. These lines are reproducible and have been included in previous works regarding headache etiology. However, when viewed through the FDM, it is often clear that a patient experiencing pain in a line that begins at a spot, ends at a spot, and is tender to touch along its length is experiencing a triggerband. Correction of the triggerband, achieved by ironing out the wrinkled tissue, can provide significant improvement in a patient's headache complaint (Figs. 6.1, 6.2 and 6.3).

Continuum distortion (CD) headaches

Continuum distortion (CD) headaches are characterized by the patient gesturing to single spots of pain, either a single spot of pain or multiple individual spots of pain. The gesture is a single finger identifying the location of pain on the bone. Correction of the CD provides relief of the headache.

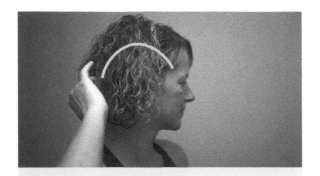

FIGURE 6.1
Scalp triggerband

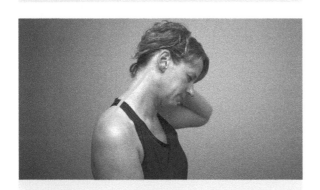

FIGURE 6.2
Shoulder–mastoid triggerband

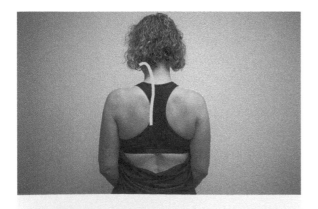

FIGURE 6.3
Star triggerband

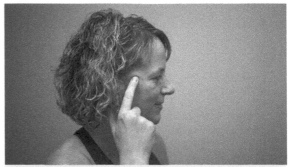

FIGURE 6.4
Temporal continuum distortion (CD)

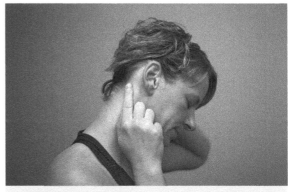

FIGURE 6.5
Occipital continuum distortion (CD)

Common locations of this type of headache and distortion in the head are temporal CDs, occipital CDs, head CDs, and supraorbital CDs (Figs. 6.4, 6.5, 6.6 and 6.7).

Herniated triggerpoints (HTPs)

The head region can have HTPs just like any other region in the body. By carefully observing the patient's gesture, the practitioner will notice that multiple fingers are used to identify the source of pain. This multi-finger gesture is consistent with an HTP in the head region.

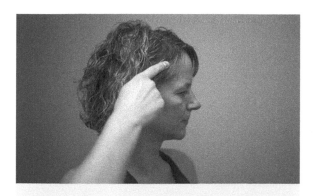

FIGURE 6.6
Head continuum distortion (CD)

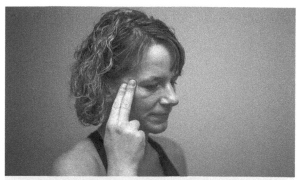

FIGURE 6.8
Temporal herniated trigger point (HTP)

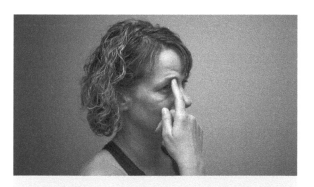

FIGURE 6.7
Supraorbital continuum distortion (CD)

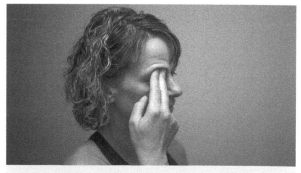

FIGURE 6.9
Supraorbital herniated trigger point (HTP)

Common locations for pain in the head region due to HTPs are the temporal, lacrimal, occipital, and maxillary region (Figs. 6.8, 6.9, 6.10, 6.11 and 6.12).

Folding distortion (FD) headaches

Headaches that seem to be located deep in the head are frequently identified by the patient grabbing and squeezing the head (Fig. 6.13). The patient will hold the head and compress in the direction providing the most relief. These are thought of as folding distortion (FD) headaches. When the patient demonstrates this type of headache, the treatment

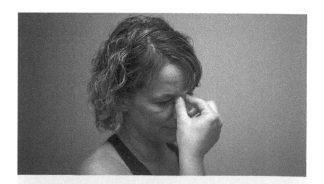

FIGURE 6.10
Lacrimal herniated trigger point (HTP)

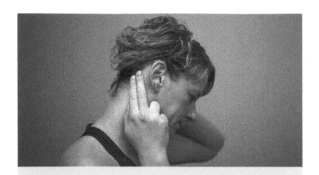

FIGURE 6.11
Occipital herniated trigger point (HTP)

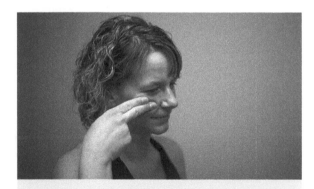

FIGURE 6.12
Maxillary herniated trigger point (HTP)

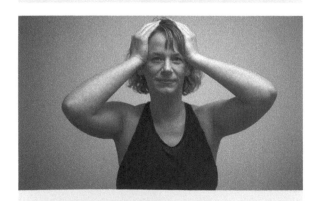

FIGURE 6.13
Folding distortion (FD) headache

is to squeeze or compress the head with the intent to refold or unfold the distorted fascia. It is important to understand that compressing (refolding) the skull in one direction will induce unfolding in the area perpendicular to the area being compressed (Fig. 6.14).

When treating a folding of the head region, the practitioner must keep in mind that the treatment should not hurt. Communicating with the patient

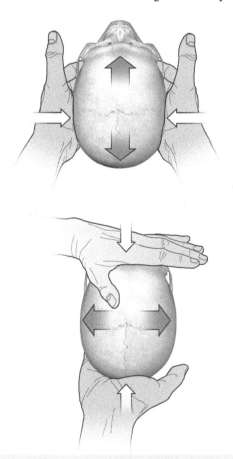

FIGURE 6.14
Refolding the skull in one direction, inducing unfolding in the area perpendicular to the area being compressed

will enable the practitioner to apply pressure in the exact direction that feels the best. In addition to static compression, a compression thrust can also be applied. Occasionally there will be an articulation deep in the skull as the head is folded. Again, this treatment should not be painful. If pain is experienced, the treatment should not be performed in that direction and the force direction adjusted until relief is felt (Figs. 6.15 and 6.16).

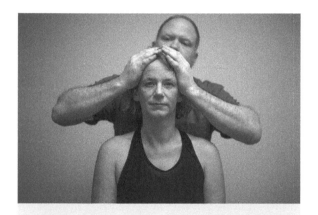

FIGURE 6.15
Folding distortion (FD) headache treatment, upright

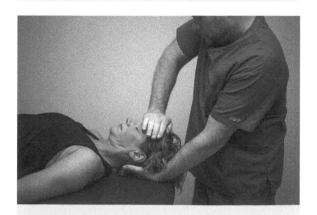

FIGURE 6.16
Folding distortion (FD) headache treatment, supine

Cylinder distortion (CyD) headaches

These are frequently bizarre or unusual headaches that are described by the patient with a sweeping motion. Frequently, the patient's hand does not touch their hair or scalp during this sweeping motion, describing their pain from a distance (Fig. 6.17). This gesture from a distance may be used to describe with a cylinder distortion (CyD) anywhere in the body. Patients may report a severe headache or a headache associated with numbness, tingling, or paresthesia, and may also complain of difficulty with word finding, confusion, dizziness/lightheadedness, anxiety, or difficulty concentrating. Patients who have gone bald as part of a natural process do not seem to develop CyD in the region of the hair loss. In contrast, patients who have shaved their head appear to be able to develop CyD. Therefore, functioning hair follicles may play a role in the formation of CyD in the head.

Treatment of this type of headache often involves pulling the hair. If the patient has hair of sufficient length, the practitioner can apply traction with the patient's hair, gently lifting the scalp from the most superficial fascial coils, allowing them to uncoil. It is

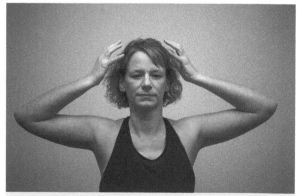

FIGURE 6.17
Sweeping at a distance

important to apply traction in such a way that does not cause undue pain (Fig. 6.18). Adjusting the grip on the hair so that traction is equal often helps reduce the "pulling hair" sensation to a sensation that is described as pleasant. A patient with a CyD headache who is being treated correctly will often intuitively know that the treatment is correct, and lean into the hair pulling. As the patient relaxes, the scalp feels as though it is pulling from the skull or as if the hair

is lengthening in the practitioner's grip. Patients can easily perform this technique at home. In patients with a shaved head, cups and other suction devices can be used to grasp the shaved skin and mobilize the most superficial fascia under the skin (Fig. 6.19).

As with any region of the body, there may be several types of distortions present in the head, each contributing to the pain complaint. By observing the patient's gestures and reassessing after each distortion is treated, significant relief can be provided to the patient.

Jaw pain

Patients frequently present with jaw pain, often accompanied by a diagnosis of temporomandibular joint (TMJ) pain whether or not the TMJ is the source of the pain. When treating the jaw, watching the midline of the upper and lower teeth and how they approximate is a helpful guide for evaluating the progress of the treatment (Fig. 6.20). In addition, observing the way a patient opens and closes the jaw and the occlusion of the teeth can help direct treatment. If a patient demonstrates a line of pain, they

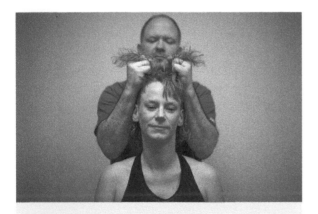

FIGURE 6.18
Hair traction for cylinder distortion (CyD) headache

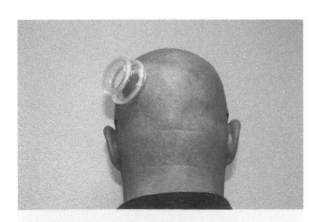

FIGURE 6.19
Cupping for cylinder distortion (CyD) headache

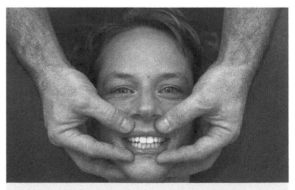

FIGURE 6.20
Monitoring approximation of the upper and lower teeth

are demonstrating a triggerband. A common trigger-band associated with jaw pain moves from the TMJ to the tip of the chin (Fig. 6.21).

Pain in the TMJ itself is often identified as a single spot of pain, signifying the presence of a CD. CDs can be found both external on the skin overlying the TMJ and internally on the inner aspect of the jaw, but as always, keep in mind that CDs occur wherever the patient indicates them (Fig. 6.22).

Some CDs are located on the origin or insertion of the pterygoid and may require treatment inside the mouth. When corrected, the patient will report decreased pain in the TMJ and normalization of function.

Very little force is usually required to reduce CDs of the TMJ. Proper technique and focused force are important for successful treatment.

FDs of the jaw or TMJ are identified when the patient holds the jaw (Fig. 6.23). This folding gesture does not identify which type of folding is present unless a line is drawn across the TMJ, at which point a rFD would be suspected.

Treatment of TMJ FDs begins with testing the patient's pain when refolding or unfolding the jaw. The history of the jaw pain, including inciting events and a description of activities which elicit pain (such as opening or closing the jaw), can provide valuable information to guide treatment. Refolding the jaw can be performed with the jaw slightly open and the teeth apart. The chin is grasped, applying pressure into the joint through

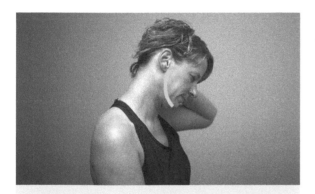

FIGURE 6.21
Jaw triggerband

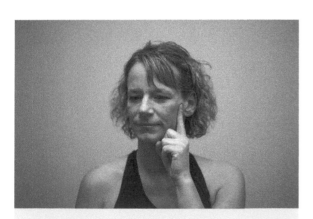

FIGURE 6.22
Temporomandibular continuum distortion (CD)

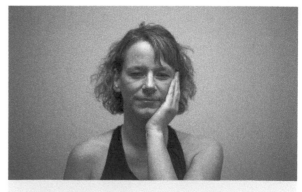

FIGURE 6.23
Jaw/temporomandibular joint (TMJ) folding distortion (FD)

the mandible (Fig. 6.24 and 6.25). The force can be applied into an individual TMJ, or it can be applied to both at the same time if this is determined to be the correct vector of treatment (Figs. 6.26 and 6.27). If this is painful, the force is reversed 180 degrees and the joint is unfolded. Unfolding can be performed in the supine position or seated position. With this treatment, the cervical spine is rotated to the side away from treatment. The patient's head

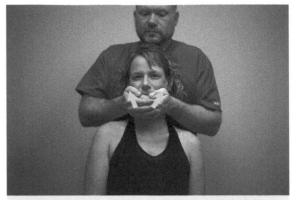

FIGURE 6.26
Bilateral jaw/temporomandibular joint (TMJ) refolding treatment, upright

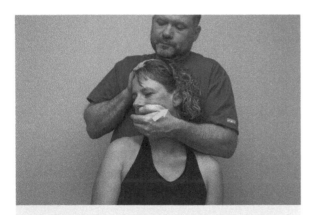

FIGURE 6.24
Jaw refolding treatment, upright

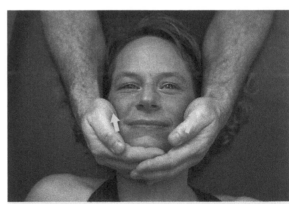

FIGURE 6.27
Bilateral jaw/temporomandibular joint (TMJ) refolding treatment, supine

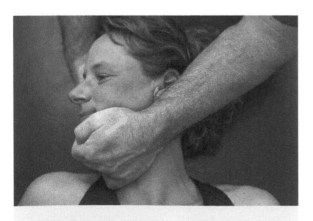

FIGURE 6.25
Jaw refolding treatment, supine

can be stabilized by the table when they are supine or against the practitioner's epigastric region or sternum when seated (Figs. 6.28 and 6.29). The heel of the hand is then placed on the angle of the jaw, and gentle pressure is applied to assess for pain. If this pressure is not painful, a thrust can be applied, making sure that the neck is locked out in rotation. If it is painful, a refolding may be present.

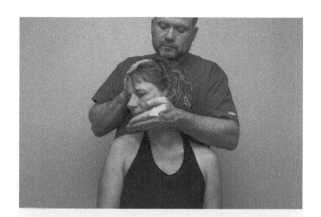

FIGURE 6.28
Jaw/temporomandibular joint (TMJ) unfolding treatment, upright

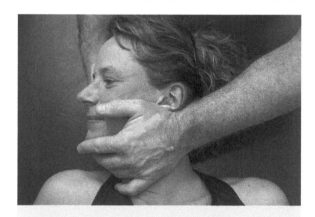

FIGURE 6.29
Jaw/temporomandibular joint (TMJ) unfolding treatment, supine

It is worth noting that the TMJ is the only joint in the body that has a rigid connection to its contralateral counterpart via the mandible. As a result, oblique forces applied to the mandible may have opposing effects for each of the TMJs. For instance, a blow to the left side of the mandible that translates the lower jaw to the right would induce an unfolding distortion (uFD) at the left TMJ, while compression induces a refolding distortion (rFD) at the right TMJ.

Decreased hearing

Dr Typaldos discussed using the auricle of the ear to apply force into the inner ear, releasing tectonically-fixed ossicles. A fast tug on the ear lobe in each direction may mobilize the ossicles, improving their function and improving hearing. When successful there is a significant audible "pop". In general, three pops can be achieved (Figs. 6.30, 6.31 and 6.32).

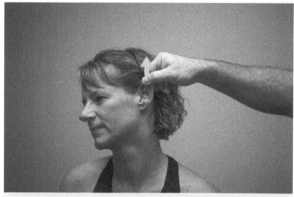

FIGURE 6.30
Ear tug, superior

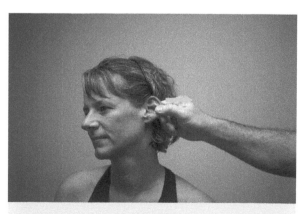

FIGURE 6.31
Ear tug, posterior

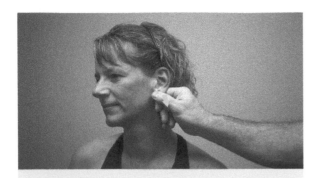

FIGURE 6.32
Ear tug, inferior

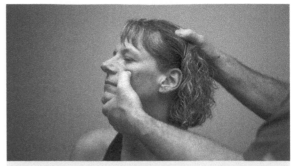

FIGURE 6.34
Maxillary herniated trigger point (HTP) treatment

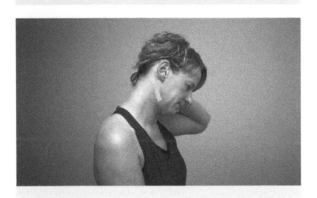

FIGURE 6.33
Triggerband associated with Eustachian tube dysfunction

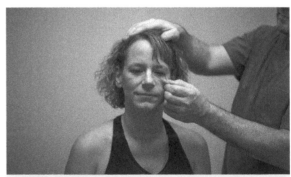

FIGURE 6.35
Skin rolling technique for cylinder distortion (CyD) treatment

Eustachian tube dysfunction

Treating CDs and triggerbands associated with the Eustachian tubes can improve drainage and overall function (Fig. 6.33).

Maxillary pain

Pain described in the maxillary sinuses is often attributed to inflammation or infection of the sinuses. The observant FDM practitioner may recognize the gesture often used to describe the maxillary pain as being consistent with an HTP of the maxillary region (Fig. 6.34). Treating the HTP in the area of the maxillary nerve can provide significant reduction of sinusitis symptoms.

Facial pain

An unusual or bizarre sensation in the face may be due to a CyD of the face. As with CyDs in other areas of the body, the pain may be unusually intense or feel as though it jumps from spot to spot around the face. Patients may also report their face feels dough-like or numb. Skin rolling is an effective technique for addressing CyDs in this region (Fig. 6.35).

As previously discussed, it is unnecessary to divide the body into regions other than for simplifying instruction on techniques. Many of the principles and treatments discussed in other sections can be used to resolve cervical region pain.

Cervical triggerbands

Triggerbands of the neck are often associated with the patient complaining their neck is stiff or tight. Patients may feel pulling when turning through the normal range of motion (ROM). When treating triggerbands in the neck, the practitioner should be aware that the superficial fascia between the skin and muscles is quite thin in this area, and so instead of pressing deep into the neck, reducing the angle of the thumb relative to the skin surface and the amount of force applied can make for a more tolerable and effective treatment.

Star triggerband

The "star of the show" is commonly associated with neck pain. This triggerband can extend up over the scalp or end at the ipsilateral mastoid. Treatment of this triggerband can dramatically improve neck pain and cervicogenic headaches (Fig. 7.1).

Posterior shoulder triggerband

Posterior shoulder triggerband begins at the elbow of one arm, progresses toward the head, crosses midline at T1 or C7, and ends at the contralateral mastoid. Although this triggerband is not confined to the cervical region, patients experiencing neck complaints may describe it (Fig. 7.2).

Anterior shoulder triggerband

This classic shoulder triggerband may be seen in patients complaining of neck pain. This triggerband

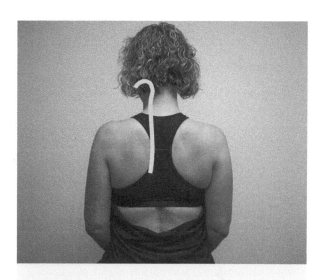

FIGURE 7.1
Star triggerband

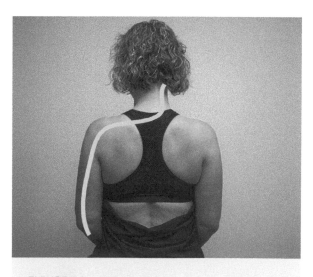

FIGURE 7.2
Posterior shoulder triggerband

begins near the elbow and travels anteriorly over the bicep. It then crosses the shoulder anterior to the tip of the acromioclavicular joint and courses across the upper shoulder into the neck, ending at the ipsilateral mastoid (Fig. 7.3).

Sternocleidomastoid triggerband

Patients experiencing tightness in the front of the neck during rotation, flexion, or extension may show a line of pain in the region of the sternocleidomastoid muscle (SCM). This triggerband is often superficial and so treatment requires attention to the underlying anatomical structures of the neck and careful application of oblique (rather than deep) force.

Shoulder–mastoid triggerband

The shoulder–mastoid triggerband is a very common in patients complaining of neck pain. It can be associated with tightness and pulling in many ROMs.

As with all triggerbands, the origin and insertion of the triggerband may have an associated continuum distortion (CD), in this case at either the occiput or the acromioclavicular joint (Fig. 7.4).

Pericervical triggerband

Multiple triggerbands on the dorsal aspect of the neck may be present, similar to the path of the star triggerband. Slight variations in the route of the triggerband from the shoulder to the spine may exist. Multiple pericervical triggerbands can be present in patients with severe neck tightness, for example in a whiplash scenario.

Cervical herniated trigger points (HTPs)

HTPs occur wherever the patient identifies them. HTPs in this region often contribute to decreased rotation of the cervical spine as well as the abduction of the shoulder.

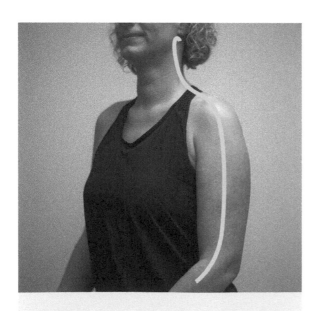

FIGURE 7.3
Anterior shoulder triggerband

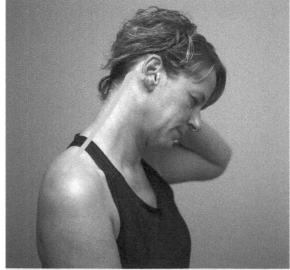

FIGURE 7.4
Shoulder-mastoid triggerband

Supraclavicular HTP (SCHTP)

The SCHTP is one of the most prevalent HTPs in the body. Besides the patient gesture, this HTP frequently presents with radicular pain and pain associated with altered sensation in the hand.

Anterior SCHTP

These HTPs are located superior to the clavicle and anterior to the midline of the body. They are commonly associated with the large vascular and nerve structures in this region. Careful attention to the method and force of treatment is essential. In this area, the direction of force applied for treatment is much more important than the amount of force. This HTP can be very painful to reduce. Careful attention to technique can improve patient tolerance and effectiveness of treatment (Fig. 7.5).

Posterior SCHTP

This is the most common form of SCHTP and is regarded as the number-one loss of abduction of the shoulder, internal rotation of the shoulder, and rotation of the cervical spine. It is a frequent source of discomfort in patients who work for long periods at a desk or on a computer. Reduction of posterior HTP can be complicated due to the many layers of overlapping fascia in the region. Patient positioning can simplify reduction of this HTP, and practitioner body mechanics are important when attempting to reduce all HTPs (Figs. 7.6, 7.7 and 7.8).

Occipital HTP

The observant FDM practitioner will notice that the occiput is often identified as the location of neck pain. The patient's hair may obscure the exact location of the distortion and number of fingers used

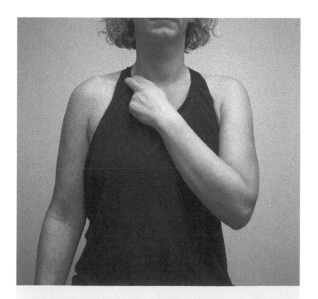

FIGURE 7.5
Anterior supraclavicular herniated triggerpoint (HTP)

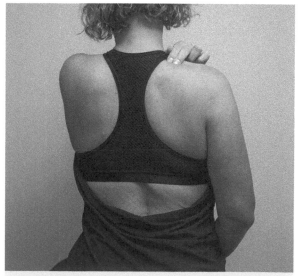

FIGURE 7.6
Posterior supraclavicular herniated triggerpoint (HTP)

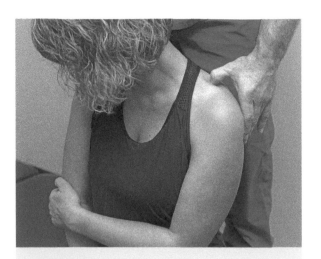

FIGURE 7.7
Supraclavicular herniated triggerpoint (HTP) treatment, seated

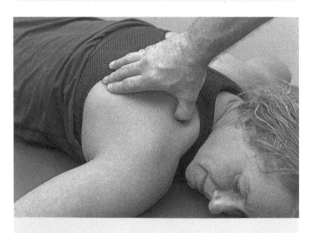

FIGURE 7.8
Supraclavicular herniated triggerpoint (HTP) treatment, prone

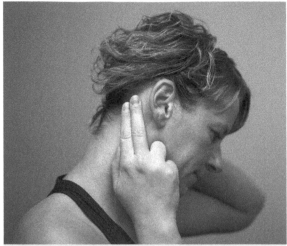

FIGURE 7.9
Occipital herniated triggerpoint (HTP)

to indicate the painful area, requiring additional care when observing gestures in this region. Two fingers or a thumb pressed into the occipital region indicates an HTP in this area (Fig. 7.9), while a single finger indicates a continuum distortion (CD), see below.

Cervical continuum distortions (CDs)

Continuum distortions (CDs) occur wherever the patient identifies them. These distortions represent a disruption of the fascial/bone continuum. Correcting the disrupted mechanism at the fascial bone intersection will reset the continuum and provide relief.

Occipital CD

A single finger pointing or pressing into the occiput or occipital region indicates a CD (Fig. 7.10).

Spinous process CD

Any spinal vertebra can have a CD of the spinous process. Patients will gesture with a single finger pointing to the vertebra of the neck. The practitioner will be guided to the exact spot of pain by the patient's gesture (Fig. 7.11).

Transverse process CD

The cervical vertebra may develop single, discrete spots of pain on the articular pillar or transverse process.

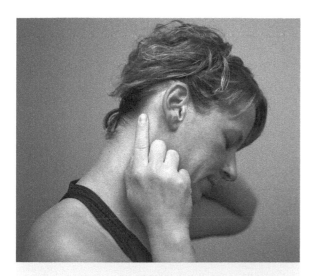

FIGURE 7.10
Occipital continuum distortion (CD)

The areas of pain identified with a single finger represent CDs of the cervical vertebra (Fig. 7.12).

Clavicular CD

Patients with neck pain may identify individual tender points along the clavicle. These tender points can be associated with loss of ROM in the cervical spine as well as the shoulder. These points may represent the disrupted fascia–bone connection at the end of the banded fascia. Patients will identify these individual spots of pain with a single finger (Fig. 7.13).

Cervical folding distortions (FDs)

Patients experiencing folding distortions (FDs) of the cervical region will hold the neck or a portion of the neck (Fig. 7.14). The practitioner should pay attention to what factors worsen and improve the

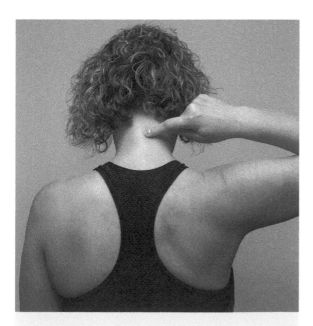

FIGURE 7.11
Spinous process continuum distortion (CD)

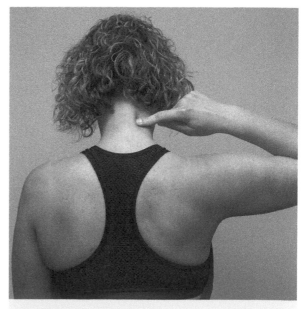

FIGURE 7.12
Transverse process continuum distortion (CD)

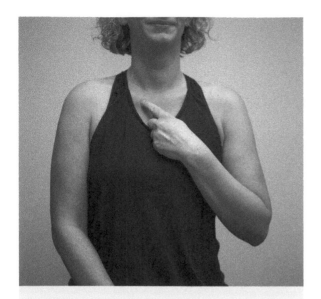

FIGURE 7.13
Clavicular continuum distortion (CD)

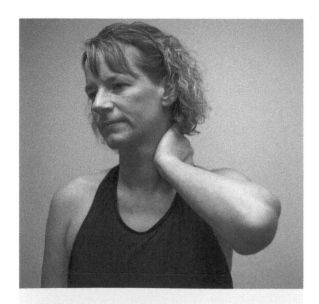

FIGURE 7.14
Cervical folding distortion (FD)

patient's neck pain, as this information can help a practitioner determine what type of folding is present and what type of folding treatment to perform in this situation. FD treatments should not hurt. If traction of the neck improves a patient's neck pain, an unfolding distortion (uFD) may be present; but if compression of the cervical spine relieves pain, then an unfolding treatment would not be appropriate, and a compressive force would need to be applied to the neck instead.

Cervical unfolding distortions (uFDs)

Unfolding treatment of the cervical spine is performed with axial traction. If a patient is complaining of neck pain, and this pain feels better in the morning or with traction, then a supine unfolding of the cervical spine can be performed.

With this technique, the patient lays supine on a treatment table while the practitioner cups one hand under the occiput and one hand over the patient's chin. The patient's chin is directed to cervical neutral, which is often with the chin slightly downward, then gently applies traction force. If this is not painful, a cephalad thrust can be applied (Fig. 7.15).

Cervical refolding distortions (rFDs)

Refolding distortions (rFDs) in the cervical region are associated with pain that improves throughout the day or improves with compression. Besides the gesture of holding the neck, the patient may draw a line across the neck (Fig. 7.16). In this case, a refolding of the cervical spine should be performed.

Refolding of the cervical spine can be performed by placing compressive force onto the cervical region through an axial load. The practitioner applies compressive force to the neck by placing their hands on the head while seated or laying down, directing the force through the head, compressing the neck.

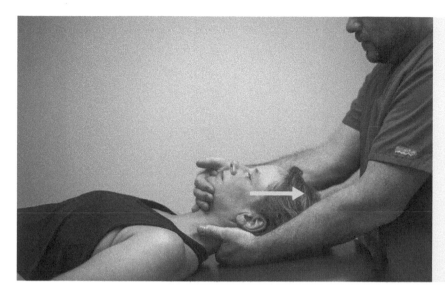

FIGURE 7.15
Cervical unfolding distortion (uFD) treatment

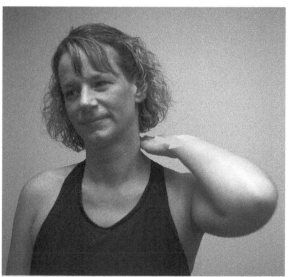

FIGURE 7.16
Cervical refolding distortion (rFD) patient gesture

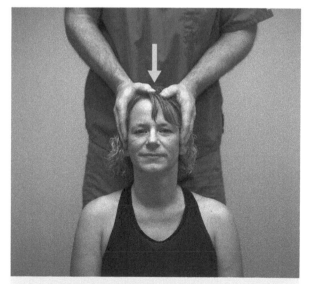

FIGURE 7.17
Cervical refolding distortion (rFD) treatment, seated

The practitioner should feel the neck compressing. If compression stops and the patient is still not experiencing pain, slight rotation of the cervical spine may allow additional compression of the cervical spine to be achieved. Each vertebral level may require subtle rotational adjustments for compression to be successful. When the cervical spine feels completely compressed, treatment is complete and the cervical spine is allowed to return to neutral by rapidly releasing the compression (Fig. 7.17).

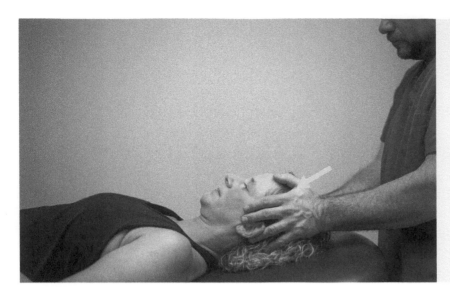

FIGURE 7.18
Cervical refolding distortion (rFD) treatment, supine

Alternately, this treatment can be performed with the patient supine on the treatment table. The practitioner adjusts the table to place the patient's head at the same level as the practitioner's epigastric region, allowing the practitioner to grasp the edges of the table and apply a compression of the cervical spine with their epigastric region. Constant force can be applied with practitioner body movement providing the subtle adjustments required to refold the cervical spine completely. Thoracic spine refolding may also be performed with this technique (Fig. 7.18).

Cervical high-velocity, low-amplitude (HVLA) with unfolding and refolding

Cervical thrust manipulation, or high-velocity, low-amplitude (HVLA) manipulation, is a technique taught in many types of manual therapy. If the technique is already in the practitioner's toolbox and within their scope of practice, incorporating FDM into cervical thrust manipulation can add a new dimension to treatment.

HVLA of the cervical vertebra requires the practitioner to assess individual spinal segments for flexion, extension, rotation, and side bending. When adding the FDM to the HVLA technique, the practitioner additionally assesses whether a uFD or rFD is present in the segment to be treated through patient history, mechanism of injury, or by actual testing while maneuvering the cervical spine. By considering the unfolding and refolding element of the cervical vertebral segment, the practitioner can induce this axial refolding or unfolding during the HVLA maneuver. If the practitioner keeps in mind that treatment of an rFD and uFD does not hurt, the treatment will not be painful. Adding refolding or unfolding may be the key to reducing or eliminating pain that some patients feel with traditional HVLA (Figs. 7.19 and 7.20).

Still technique with folding in mind

The Still technique easily incorporates into the Fascial Distortion Model, visualized as treating FDs. Using compression and traction forces to follow a joint's movement allows the practitioner to refold and unfold those joints. By applying the unfolding and refolding mechanism to the fascial matrix while performing Still technique, the practitioner can

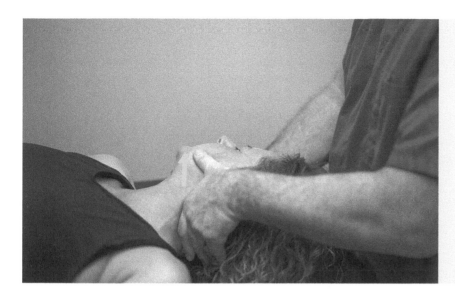

FIGURE 7.19
Cervical high-velocity,
low-amplitude (HVLA) with
unfolding vector

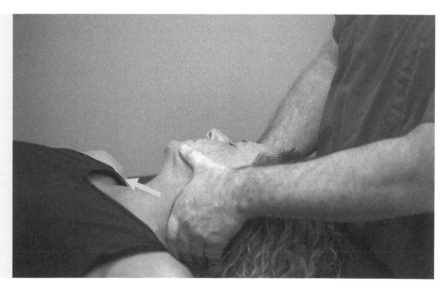

FIGURE 7.20
Cervical high-velocity,
low-amplitude (HVLA) with
refolding vector

better visualize their treatment, which may enhance their effectiveness.

Cervical cylinder distortions (CyDs)

Cylinder distortions (CyDs) in the cervical region are associated with bizarre and unusual pain. Tingling, nerve-like pain may be present, which can be confused for discogenic problems. The patient with CyD may gesture by repetitively squeezing the neck or sweeping along the neck. The pain may jump from one place to another and can be of inexplicable intensity.

Many cylinder techniques can be used to treat CyD of the neck. When treating CyD in this area, attention should be paid to the underlying neuro-vascular structures, and the practitioner should also recall that the affected fascia in this region is often very superficial. Treatment of this superficial fascia does not require much force to achieve separation of the tangled coils of fascia (Fig. 7.21).

Double-thumb technique

Double-thumb technique can treat CyD in the cervical region. Again, one must pay attention so that compression of the carotid body does not occur while correcting CyD (Fig. 7.22).

Squeegee technique

The posterior aspect of the neck can be treated effectively with the squeegee technique.

Cupping with movement

Cupping with movement can be a very effective technique for addressing CyDs of the cervical spine, especially useful for complaints that include distortions over the upper trapezius. Cups are usually placed where the patient demonstrates the distortion, with the size and the number of cups determined by watching the patient's gesture and matching the size of the cup to the size and number of areas identified by the patient (Fig. 7.23). Once the cup is placed, the patient moves their neck and arms through a ROM.

Cervical tectonic fixations (TFs)

When a patient is experiencing a tectonic fixation (TF) in the cervical spine, they rarely have an accompanying gesture to identify this distortion, but they may have overlying distortions present that do have gestures associated with them. By paying careful attention to the patient's history and the description of their pain, the practitioner can identify TFs of the cervical spine in the presence of other distortions.

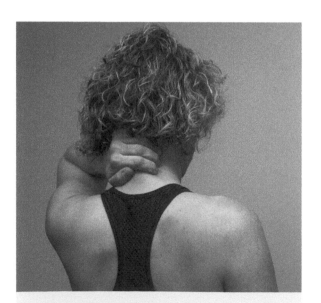

FIGURE 7.21
Cervical cylinder distortion (CyD) "squeezing" gesture

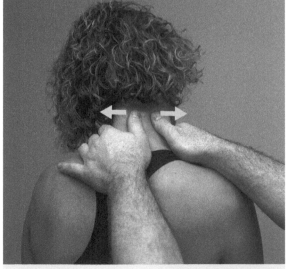

FIGURE 7.22
Double-thumb technique for cervical cylinder distortion (CyD)

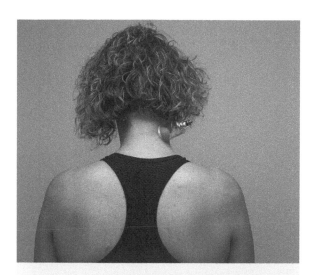

FIGURE 7.23
Cupping for cervical cylinder distortion (CyD)

These patients often have the feeling that their cervical spine needs to be cracked and often use their own hands to add force to rotation and side bending of their cervical spine to induce movement. These patients may find much relief with the application of heat before treatment.

HVLA technique

The HVLA maneuvers discussed earlier in this section are also very effective at addressing TFs of the cervical spine Applying heat before treatment of TF may improve the practitioner's ability to mobilize the cervical spine and patients who get relief with the application of heat to any portion of the body can be encouraged to do so, providing the heat is associated with, or followed by, movement and use of the area.

As with all areas of the body discussed in this text, the distortions identified are common and each distortion can extend well beyond the anatomical boundaries identified. The techniques to treat the distortions shown may be appropriately used when working with this region or for other complaints.

Thoracic triggerbands

Star triggerband

This extremely common triggerband has a powerful impact on complaints in the thoracic region. Correct treatment is important to relieve pain and tightness in this area. The triggerband generally begins at the level of T6 and runs cephalad, parallel to the thoracic spine. The fascia overlying the paraspinal musculature is a common location for this triggerband, but extension past the occiput over the skull is not uncommon, especially in patients presenting with headaches (Fig. 8.1).

Scapular triggerband

A triggerband that outlines the edge or margin of the scapula is referred to as the scapular triggerband. This triggerband generally forms a U-shape as it traces the boundaries of the scapula. Complaints of pulling, burning, or tightness may accompany patient gesture indicating this triggerband, but some patients may not be able to gesture in this region and instead rely on a verbal description or identify the location of the triggerband on someone else (Fig. 8.2).

Rib triggerband

Each rib in the thoracic region can have triggerbands associated with the fascial and muscular covering.

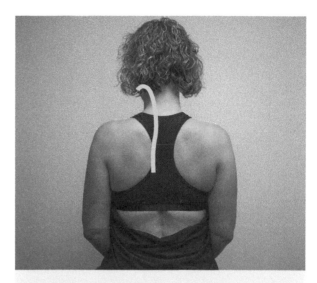

FIGURE 8.1
Star triggerband

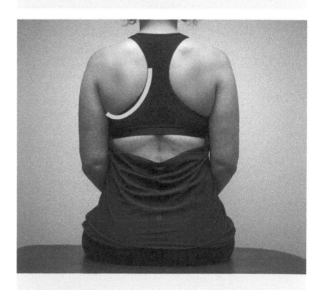

FIGURE 8.2
Scapular triggerband

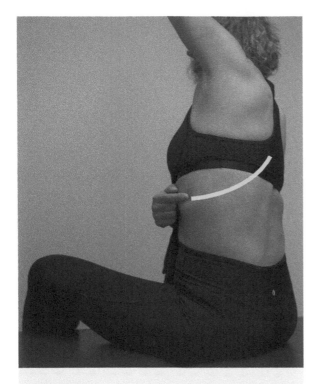

FIGURE 8.3
Rib triggerband

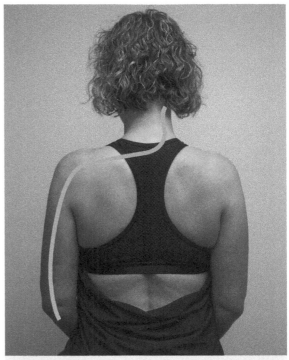

FIGURE 8.4
Posterior shoulder triggerband

It is not unusual for patient gestures to begin near a specific level on the thoracic spine and then travel laterally, approximating the pathway associated with a specific rib or rib space. The patient often describes a pulling or burning pain along that particular level (Fig. 8.3).

Posterior shoulder triggerband

This common shoulder triggerband begins below the elbow and travels posteriorly along the arm, crossing posterior to the tip of the shoulder, then crosses the upper portion of the thoracic region at the level of T1 or C7, finishing at the contralateral mastoid. The association of this triggerband with the upper portion of the thoracic region makes it a relatively common finding in patients complaining of thoracic pain (Fig. 8.4).

Anterior chest triggerband

Generally associated with the tissue overlying the pectoral muscles, patients will demonstrate this triggerband by sweeping their fingers across the upper portion of the chest.

Scapular spine triggerband

Another triggerband associated with the scapula follows the general course of the scapular spine. This triggerband is not precisely associated with the bony anatomy of the scapular spine, but rather the overlying soft tissue. It often begins in the paraspinal region of

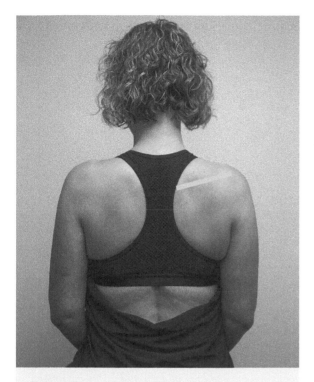

FIGURE 8.5
Scapular spine triggerband

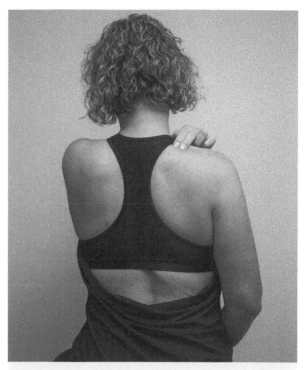

FIGURE 8.6
Supraclavicular herniated trigger point (HTP)

T4 and extends laterally toward the tip of the shoulder, crossing the region of the scapular spine (Fig. 8.5).

Thoracic herniated trigger points (HTPs)

This region of the body is prone to developing HTPs. Again, the fascial hiatus around the superficial cutaneous nerves is considered to be the focus for the formation of most HTPs. The thoracic region has an abundance of cutaneous nerve bundles, as well as some that extend caudally from the neck. HTPs occur wherever the patient demonstrates them.

Supraclavicular HTP (SCHTP)

Often when a patient presents with pain in the thoracic region, they will identify the SCHTP

as the source of part, if not all, of their pain (Fig. 8.6).

Scapulothoracic HTP

Patients with thoracic pain accompanied by shoulder pain will often present with pain at the location of the scapulothoracic joint. The area around T4 is commonly identified as a cause of pain with a gesture of multiple fingers pressing into the soft tissue (Fig. 8.7). Treatment of this HTP is often crucial in relieving the complaint of thoracic back pain. It may be helpful to have the patient place the back of their hand on their low back to wing the scapula and remove the medial edge from the area of treatment. HTPs in the upper thoracic region that appear

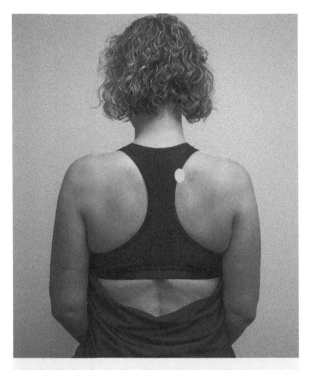

FIGURE 8.7
Scapulothoracic herniated trigger point (HTP)

to originate between the posterior ribs may benefit from positioning with the upper body flexed at the level of pain, using a therapy ball, treatment table, or with the patient hunching over to accentuate flexion at the level of pain (Fig. 8.8).

Intercostal HTP

These HTPs occur anywhere in the region of the ribs identified by the patient. Patients commonly refer to this pain as thoracic back pain. The pain is demonstrated with multiple fingers or a thumb pressing between the ribs. Reduction of these HTPs can be hastened using a therapy ball, treatment table, or through positioning the patient's body to maximize the separation of the ribs that the HTP has herniated through (Fig. 8.9).

Pectoral HTP

The upper portion of the pectoral muscle is often described as a source of pain and is demonstrated by the patient pressing multiple fingers into the upper pectoral muscle. This HTP is commonly reduced

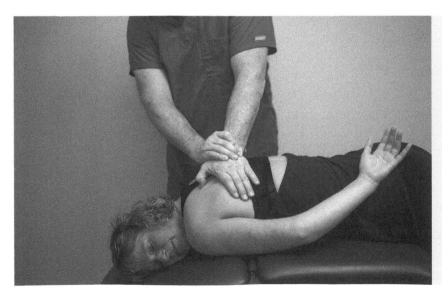

FIGURE 8.8
Scapulothoracic herniated trigger point (HTP) treatment. Note the flexion achieved by lowering the head of the treatment table.

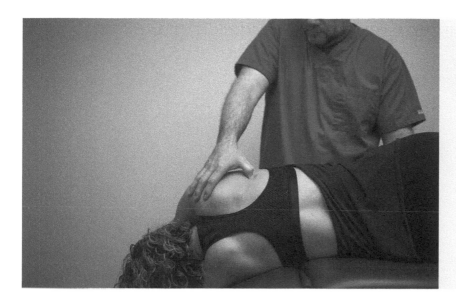

FIGURE 8.9
Intercostal herniated trigger point (HTP) treatment with sidebending

deep to the pectoral muscle and anterior to the ribs (Fig. 8.10).

Rib fascial rent

A fascial rent is a variant of an HTP, and is a large herniation of tissue through a triggerband (Fig. 8.11). The linear opening allows a significant amount of underlying fascial matrix to protrude. Traditionally, HTPs are visualized as tissue protruding up through a single, roughly circular, opening. In the thoracic region, often along the ribs, a fascial rent can occur where a triggerband of the rib forms, allowing the matrix to protrude through the triggerband. When the initial HTP is treated, there may be a firm edge identified upon palpation. The continued reduction of this edge of tissue below the fascial plane leads the practitioner to treat a linear HTP (fascial rent).

Thoracic continuum distortions (CDs)

As with all CDs, thoracic CDs occur at the fascia–bone connection anywhere a patient identifies them.

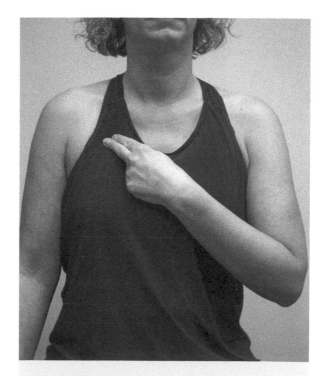

FIGURE 8.10
Pectoral herniated trigger point (HTP)

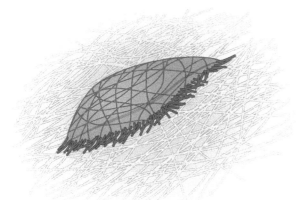

FIGURE 8.11
A fascial rent

Some common CDs have been identified and are listed below.

Spinous process CDs

The thoracic vertebra has multiple fascial connections. Like the vertebrae in other regions of the body, the attachment of the fascia to the spinous process may develop a CD (Fig. 8.12).

Transverse process CDs

These CDs are often identified by patients experiencing thoracic pain. They will use one finger to indicate their point of pain.

Costochondral junction CDs

The junction of the fascial covering of the costochondral cartilage and bone of the rib or sternum is a potential location for the formation of CDs. CDs in this region are often diagnosed as costochondritis. Correction of CDs in this location requires a very focused and careful touch as too much force applied at the junction of the cartilage and bone can cause separation of the structures. Focused treatment of

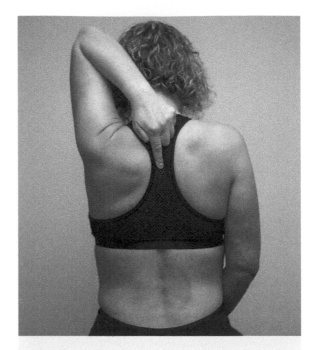

FIGURE 8.12
Spinous process continuum distortion (CD)

the fascial covering of these structures requires very little force to correct the CDs (Fig. 8.13).

Scapulothoracic CDs

CDs of the scapulothoracic joint are often identified when a patient identifies a clicking in the shoulder blade (Fig. 8.14).

Intercostal CDs

The edge of each rib has numerous fascial connections that represent continuum tissue. Disruption of the fascia–rib continuum may be the source of pinpoint pain in the ribs (Fig. 8.15).

Sternoclavicular CDs

The sternoclavicular joint and the associated fascial covering can be disrupted, leading to CDs.

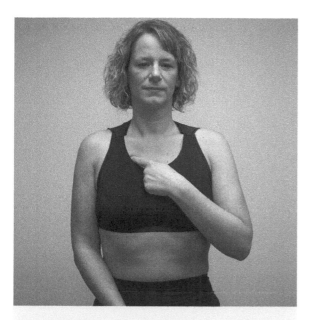

FIGURE 8.13
Costochondral junction continuum distortion (CD)

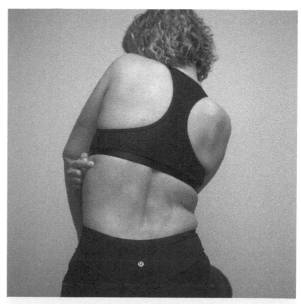

FIGURE 8.15
Intercostal continuum distortion (CD)

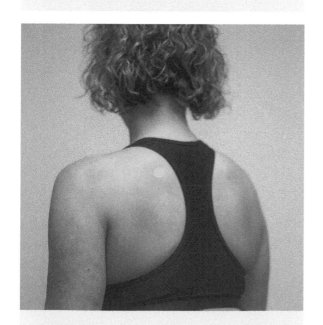

FIGURE 8.14
Scapulothoracic continuum distortion (CD)

Thoracic folding distortions (FDs)

There is a significant amount of overlapping tissue in the thoracic region. Many layers of muscle, and therefore fascia, are stacked on top of each other. Each of these layers of fascia needs to slide and glide freely for pain-free motion. The proper function of the thoracic spine folding mechanism is also critical for pain-free movement. The folding fascia of the spine is thought to behave like a shock absorber, with each vertebral level of the thoracic spine able to compress and expand, or refold and unfold, in order to absorb forces placed on the thoracic spine. Alterations to the folding fascia can prevent the normal function of the refolding/unfolding mechanism of the fascial matrix (Fig. 8.16).

Hallelujah technique

This technique is used to unfold the fascia of the thoracic vertebra. The practitioner stands behind

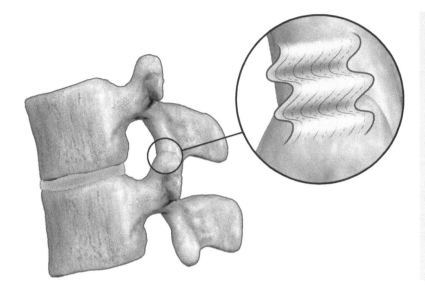

FIGURE 8.16
Thoracic folding mechanism

the patient and grasps the patient's elbows, or places their hands through the bend in the patient's arms. The patient is asked to lean against the practitioner, and the practitioner then steps backward, with their abdomen supporting the patient's thoracic region. When the patient leans back, and the abdomen is placed against the area of unfolding distortion (uFD), the patient is asked to sit down. At the same time, the provider thrusts their abdomen upwards, allowing the combination of the patient's body weight and the provider's upward thrust to separate (unfold) the thoracic vertebra. Proper use of this technique requires a match between provider and patient size. If the patient is larger than the provider, then this technique may be modified with the patient in a sitting position (Figs. 8.17, 8.18, 8.19 and 8.20).

Wall technique

In this technique, the patient faces the wall with a pillow or other soft item placed to protect the patient's head. The patient is instructed to keep their head against the wall and turned to the side. The practitioner then uses their hypothenar eminence to

engage the level of discomfort (Figs. 8.21 and 8.22) and with a firm pressure toward the overlying tissue, the thoracic region is tractioned cephalad. When the barrier is reached, a cephalad force is generated to unfold the thoracic vertebra (Fig. 8.23).

Texas Twist technique

This maneuver is used for both tectonic fixation (TF) of the thoracic region and for unfolding or refolding of the thoracic vertebra. To perform this technique, the patient lies prone on the treatment table with the practitioner's hands placed on the patient's back, one on each side of the spine. The fingers of one hand are pointing cephalad, and the fingers of the other are pointing caudad. The heels of both hands press into the soft tissue of the back, and the hands are thrust in the direction that the fingers are pointing. The hands can then be reversed so that each side of the spine is being treated in the opposite direction (Fig. 8.24).

Rib refolding distortion (rFD) treatment

The fascia between the ribs can unfold and refold. When a patient presents with a folding distortion

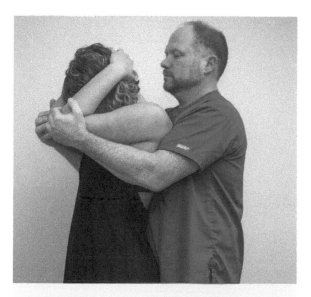

FIGURE 8.17
Hallelujah technique: positioning for thoracic unfolding distortion treatment

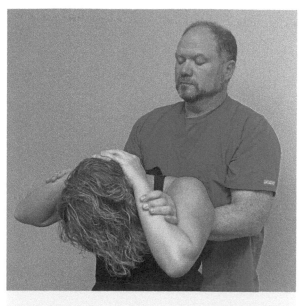

FIGURE 8.19
Hallelujah technique: alternate hand position 1

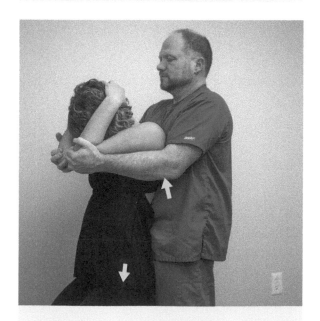

FIGURE 8.18
Hallelujah technique force vectors

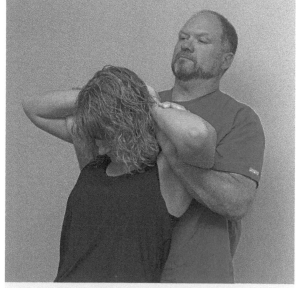

FIGURE 8.20
Hallelujah technique: alternate hand position 2

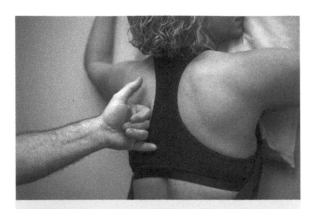

FIGURE 8.21
Hand placement 1 for thoracic unfolding wall technique

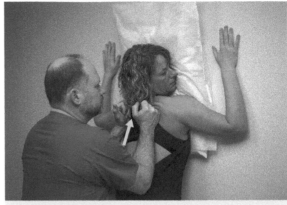

FIGURE 8.23
Wall technique force vector

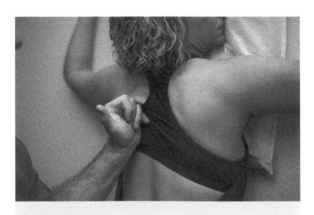

FIGURE 8.22
Hand placement 2 for thoracic unfolding wall technique

in this area, they will gesture by holding the ribs. It is important to note that this treatment should not hurt. In this technique, the practitioner's goal is to approximate two ribs, refolding the fascia between the ribs. To refold this fascia, the heel of one hand is placed on the rib (fingers pointing caudad) above the tissue needing to be refolded. The heel of the opposite hand (fingers pointing cephalad) is placed on the rib below the tissue that needs to be refolded. Both hands are on the same side of the spine. The hands are then moved toward each other. The movement should be bringing the ribs together, refolding the fascia between the ribs (Fig. 8.25).

Rib unfolding distortion (uFD) treatment

The fascia between the ribs can experience an unfolding distortion (uFD). In this situation, the tissue between the ribs needs to be separated. To unfold the fascia, the heel of one hand is placed on the superior rib to be treated with the fingers pointing cephalad. The other hand is placed on the inferior rib with the fingers pointing caudad. The hands begin on the same side of the spine, and are then separated. This treatment separates, or unfolds, the tissue between the ribs (Fig. 8.26).

Seated chair technique

This technique is used to unfold and refold the thoracic vertebra while a patient is in the seated position. Traditionally, this technique is performed

FIGURE 8.24

Texas Twist hand placement and force vectors

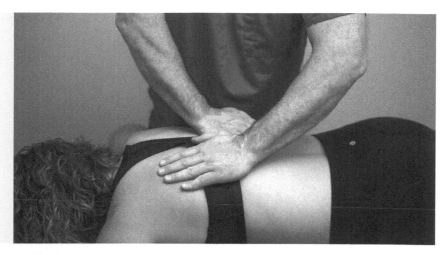

FIGURE 8.25

Rib refolding distortion (rFD) treatment

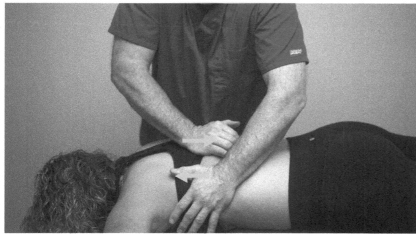

FIGURE 8.26

Rib unfolding distortion (uFD) treatment

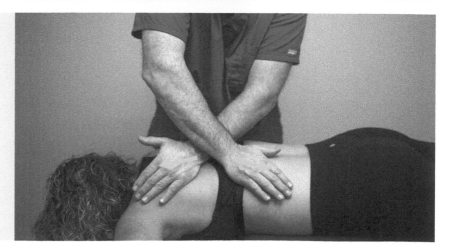

with the patient sitting backwards on a chair, placed so that their knees are pressing against a wall. They are then asked to cross their arms in front of them, grasping their shoulders. The practitioner grasps their arms with one hand, inducing rotation and side bending as needed. When treating a uFD, the patient is rotated away from the side being treated. The thenar eminence of the hand is used to accentuate an unfolding motion by thrusting upward on the ribs (Fig. 8.27). When treating a refolding distortion (rFD) with this technique, the patient is rotated away from the side being treated with little or no side bending away from the side being treated. A refolding force is applied to the thoracic spine with the thenar eminence of the hand thrusting downward (Fig. 8.28). This technique can

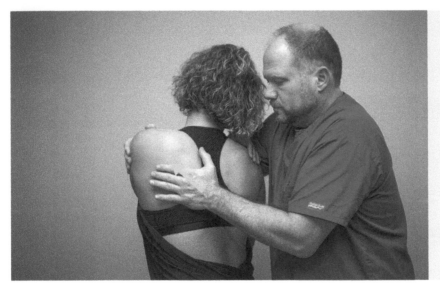

FIGURE 8.27
Chair unfolding distortion (uFD) treatment

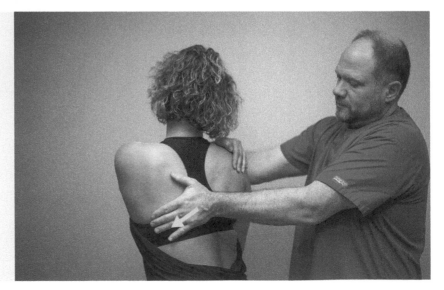

FIGURE 8.28
Chair refolding distortion (rFD) treatment

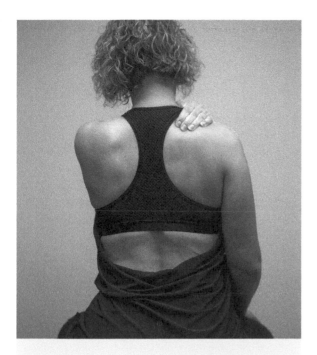

FIGURE 8.29
First rib refolding distortion (rFD): patient gesture

be adapted for use in clinic, where a patient straddles the treatment table.

First rib refolding

When a patient places the palm of their hand over the top of the shoulder, this could represent the gesture for a first rib rFD (Fig. 8.29). This gesture is in the same general area of the much more common SCHTP. Careful observation of the gesture, and differentiating between folding and HTP body language, will decrease the chance of mistaking this diagnosis. Recall that the patient will identify a painful spot if this is an HTP, and the practitioner can elicit this pain if they press on the spot. Likewise, applying pressure to a folding distortion will not be painful.

If the gesture and complaint suggest an FD of the first rib, then this can be treated by placing the patient prone on a treatment table. The practitioner then stands at the head of the table, in line with the patient's axial spine or slightly off to the side being treated, and asks the patient to turn their head

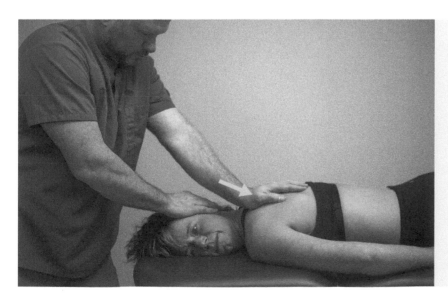

FIGURE 8.30
First rib refolding distortion (rFD) treatment

toward the side of discomfort. One hand is placed on the head while the other hypothenar eminence is placed on the first rib. The practitioner's arms should cross when in the proper setup. The hand that is resting on the patient's head does not press or move the head; it is solely for stabilization. Gently test by compressing the first rib. If no pain is present with testing, then the hand that is on the rib

compresses, taking up the slack in the movement of the first rib. When a barrier is reached, a thrust is performed in the caudal direction (Fig. 8.30).

Thoracic cylinder distortions (CyDs)

Unusual or bizarre symptoms should trigger the thought of a possible cylinder distortion (CyD). Patients with CyDs often demonstrate a sweeping

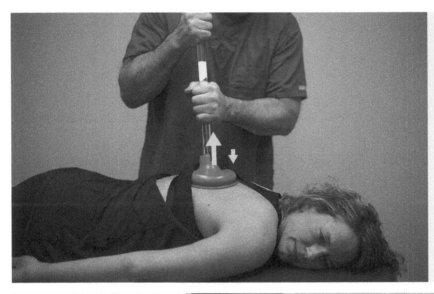

FIGURE 8.31
Plunger technique

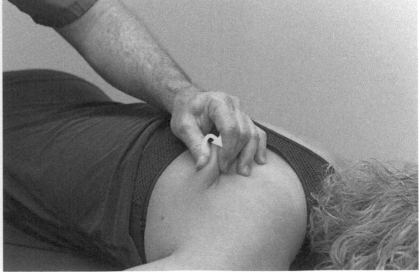

FIGURE 8.32
Skin rolling technique

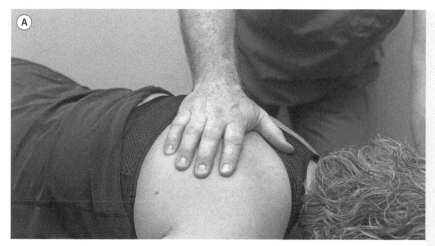

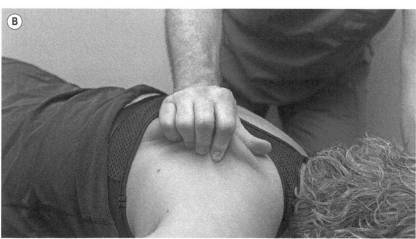

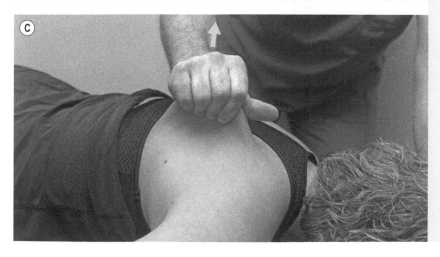

FIGURE 8.33
A–C Thoracic tiger claw technique: hand placement

or squeezing motion or report symptoms jumping from one place to another. As with all cylinder treatments, the uncoiling of the superficial cylindrical fascia should be performed. Many of the cylinder techniques uncoil the superficial coils by either stabilizing the coils and having a patient move a part of their body, or by pulling the skin away from the superficial fascia, allowing the coils to untangle.

Plunger technique

The plunger can be used to pull large sections of the thoracic skin from the underlying superficial coils. This tool is an excellent choice to consider when a patient demonstrates a large area of the body affected by the cylinder distortion (Fig. 8.31).

Skin rolling technique

This technique, which involves lifting and rolling smaller segments of the skin, can be used when a small area of CyD is identified. It can be useful for any size CyD, but due to the amount of effort required by a practitioner to treat a large cylinder with this technique, it is usually reserved for smaller areas of distortion (Fig. 8.32).

Tiger claw technique

When a patient has identified a CyD, and they have the correct skin type, the tiger claw or tiger grip technique can be used to pull the skin from the underlying coils. This technique is correctly performed by using the whole hand to grasp the skin of a patient. The hand is placed flat on the patient's skin, then closed, grasping the skin and wrapping it into the fingers. When done correctly, a firm and painless grip on the skin is achieved. It should be noted that not all patients have skin that is pliable enough to be lifted in this manner. If the skin is not pliable enough, an alternative technique should be used to address the cylinder (Fig. 8.33).

Cupping with motion

In the thoracic region, one or more cups can be placed in the area identified as a CyD. Once in place, the patient is instructed to move through a range of motion (ROM) to mobilize the fascia underlying the skin (Fig. 8.34).

Squeegee technique

Like other areas where the squeegee technique is performed, the whole surface of the hand along the first finger and thumb is used to sweep along the surface of the skin. This essentially pushes the coils out of the fascial matrix. This technique can cover broad areas with the practitioner using long sweeping treatments (Fig. 8.35).

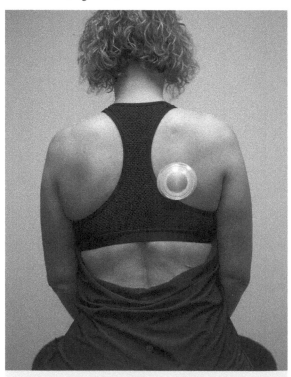

FIGURE 8.34
Thoracic cupping with motion

Thoracic tectonic fixations (TFs)

Wall technique

The wall technique, as described earlier in this section, can be used to treat TFs in the thoracic spine.

Seated chair technique

The seated chair technique that is described in the FDs section of this chapter can also be used to treat TFs of the thoracic region. When using this technique to treat TFs, the vector of treatment accentuates the rotation of the thoracic spine, and there is much less emphasis placed on the unfolding/refolding of the vertebra (Fig. 8.36).

Kirksville Crunch (double arm thrust)

This classic osteopathic high-velocity low-amplitude (HVLA) maneuver can be used to treat TFs of the thoracic spine and posterior rib heads. With this

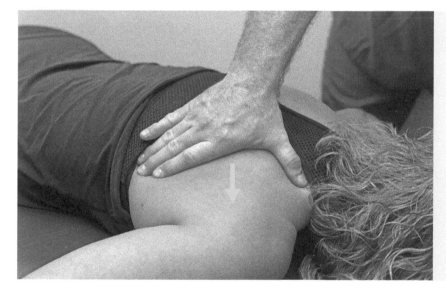

FIGURE 8.35
Thoracic squeegee technique

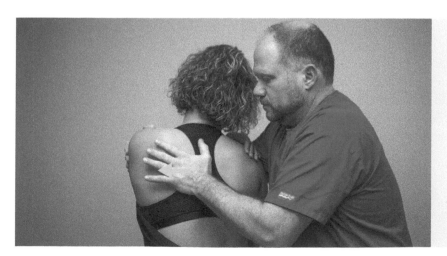

FIGURE 8.36
Chair technique for tectonic fixation (TF)

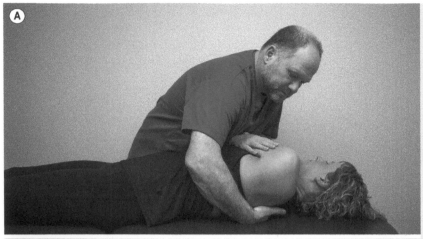

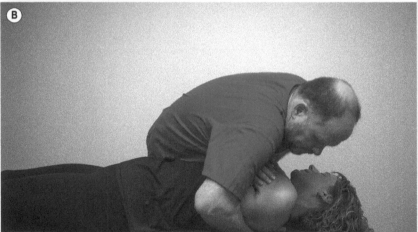

FIGURE 8.37A, B
Thoracic high-velocity, low-amplitude (HVLA) hand placement for tectonic fixation (TF)

technique, the patient lies supine on the table, with the practitioner placing the thenar eminence of the treating hand on the rib head near the spine. The patient is then rolled onto the treatment hand, forcing the rib heads back into position. While this technique can be used with a fair amount of force, it is not necessary to apply a powerful thrust to move the rib heads into position. Generally, if the practitioner is finding that the rib heads are not moving with gentle force, and the patient is still complaining of something being stuck in that region, looking for and addressing CDs and triggerbands around the rib heads will often allow the TF to resolve (Fig. 8.37).

The entire length of the spine can be treated within the Fascial Distortion Model (FDM). Many existing techniques from various manipulative modalities can be used by practitioners to treat distortions in this region, adapted to the different anatomical model or thought process of the FDM; visualizing how the technique is addressing the fascia or distortion of the fascia.

By observing patient gestures and listening to the patient, the FDM can be applied to back pain. Low back pain has far-reaching causes and implications, so in the first instance, a quality neurologic exam is important to rule out important conditions for which diagnosis and treatment should not be delayed. After completing the appropriate examination and ruling out urgent or emergent conditions, distortions can be identified and treated.

Triggerbands

Lumbar triggerbands

Lumbar triggerbands occur wherever the patient identifies them on their body; however, some common triggerbands are regularly seen and treated. Lumbar triggerbands can be parallel or perpendicular to the spine. Those that parallel the spine may start as low as the sacroiliac (SI) joint or tip of the coccyx and can extend up along the spine to the level of T6, where they may blend into the star triggerband, creating the lumbar star triggerband. Lumbar triggerbands often occur bilaterally and equidistant from the spinous process (Fig. 9.1).

> It is not uncommon to imagine this triggerband is present in the paraspinal musculature, and indeed it may be found there. However, it is important for the practitioner to remember that the distortion may be superficial to the muscles and only present in the soft tissue fascial matrix.

Lumbar triggerbands can also be identified perpendicular to the spine. The patient gesture identifying this distortion is often a line drawn laterally from the spine towards the hip (Fig. 9.2). As with all triggerbands, the lumbar triggerband is located exactly where a patient gestures, and that is where the treatment should be applied. Remember that the

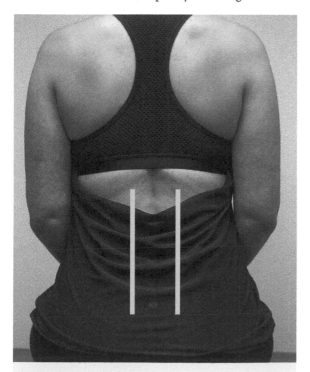

FIGURE 9.1
Lumbar triggerbands

patient may identify only a portion of a triggerband, and so the practitioner should keep common pathways in mind to improve treatment outcomes and the complete closure of the triggerband. However, it is important not to become so focused on a common pathway that the patient's body language is ignored, as this will lead to treatment failure.

If a line is drawn from one side of the lumbar spine all the way across the low back, this gesture may not be a triggerband, but rather a refolding of the lumbar spine. The differentiation can be made by listening to the patient's verbal description and attempting to treat a triggerband in the area identified. If the line being treated is not painful along its entire length, then a refolding distortion (rFD) should be considered (Fig. 9.3).

Posterior thigh triggerband

The posterior thigh triggerband is commonly demonstrated in patients experiencing low back pain. This triggerband often begins along the ipsilateral SI joint, runs superiorly towards the iliac crest, often traveling inferior to the iliac crest, then angles down the posterior aspect of the thigh. The course of the triggerband often resembles the shape of a cane (Fig. 9.4).

Lateral thigh triggerband

Another triggerband commonly demonstrated in patients experiencing back pain is the lateral thigh triggerband. This triggerband generally begins along the iliac crest, travels laterally towards the iliotibial (IT) band, and then down the leg along the IT band.

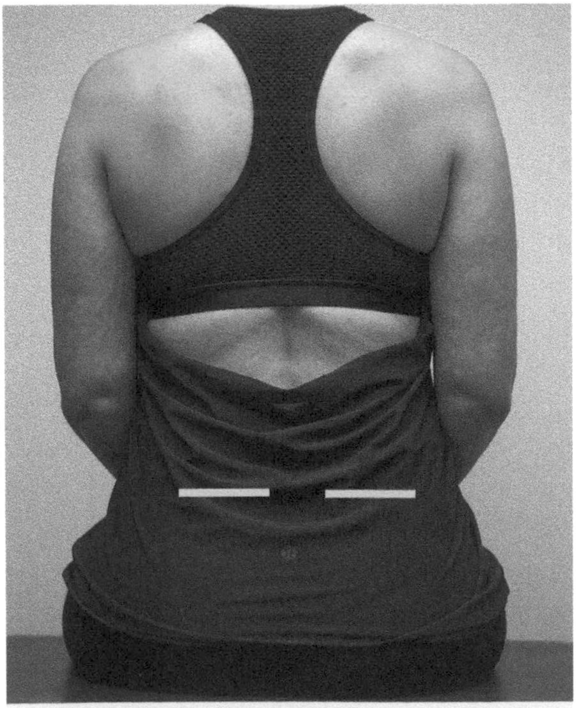

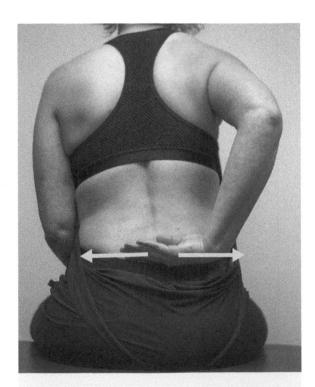

FIGURE 9.2
Lumbar triggerbands perpendicular to spine

FIGURE 9.3
Lumbar refolding distortion (rFD)

This triggerband may be directly overlying the IT band, part of the IT band, or even slightly posterior to the actual IT band. It exists precisely where the patient demonstrates (Fig. 9.5).

Lumbar herniated triggerpoints (HTPs)

This distortion is incredibly common when patients are experiencing back pain. They may use their thumb, knuckle, or fist to push into the area of pain. This distortion is found wherever the patient demonstrates it.

Lumbar HTP

This HTP is often identified when the patient presses their thumb into their low back (Fig. 9.6). They may complain of aching, especially at night. Patients often remember the event that caused the formation of the HTP, sometimes with surprising specificity and detail. This distortion is thought to last until reduced; thus it may have been present for a very long time. Patients may obtain some pain relief by pressing on the HTP themselves and it is not uncommon

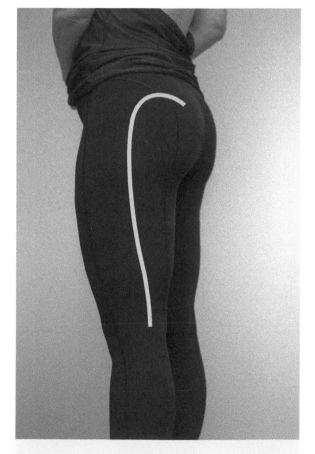

FIGURE 9.4
Posterior thigh triggerband

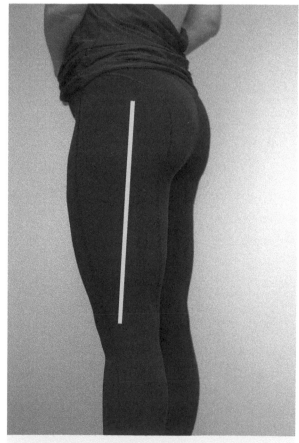

FIGURE 9.5
Lateral thigh triggerband

for patients to use a tool or have a friend or partner push on the spot for them.

Lumbar HTPs occur in the soft tissue of the lower back. The origin of HTPs is thought to be related to superficial cutaneous nerve bundles creating pathways within the fascial matrix for tissue from a deeper part of the matrix to herniate up along superficial cutaneous neurovascular complexes. Radicular pain down the leg is not uncommon when this HTP is pressing on the superficial nerve. When a patient complains of bilateral lumbar HTPs, these distortions are rarely at the same level of the body (Fig. 9.7). Treatment may be performed with the patient prone on a treatment table, standing, seated and flexed, or in child's pose (Figs. 9.8 and 9.9) and correction can provide significant rapid relief and improved ROM.

Flank HTP

Flank HTP is found in the area of the kidney. This distortion is more superior and lateral than the typical lumbar HTP. Treatment can be performed in any of the positions described as for a lumbar HTP (Fig. 9.10).

Posterior superior iliac spine (PSIS) HTP

A posterior superior iliac spine (PSIS) HTP is often found just lateral to the PSIS. Patients will often gesture with their thumb into the soft tissue

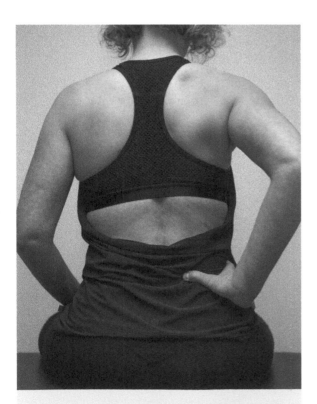

FIGURE 9.6
Lumbar herniated trigger point (HTP) patient gesture

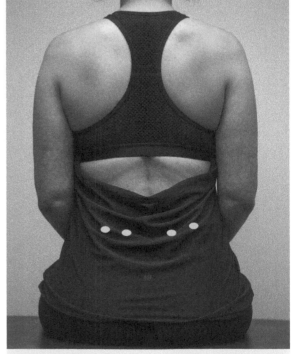

FIGURE 9.7
Common lumbar herniated trigger point (HTP) locations

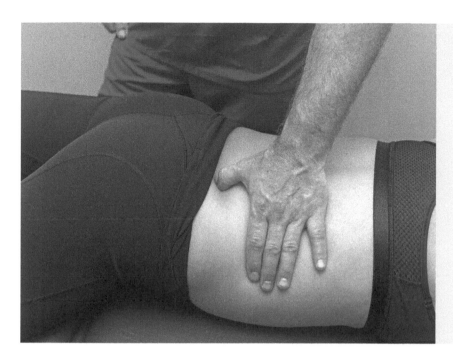

FIGURE 9.8
Lumbar herniated trigger
point (HTP) treatment, prone

FIGURE 9.9
Lumbar herniated trigger
point (HTP) treatment, child's
pose

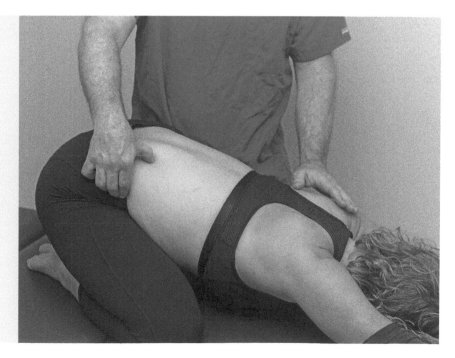

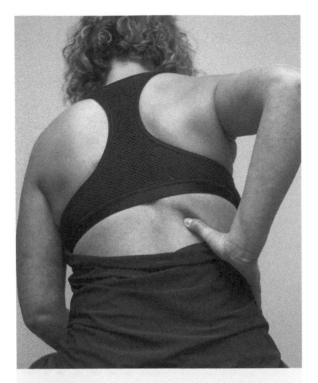

FIGURE 9.10
Flank herniated trigger point (HTP) patient gesture

and speak of trying to reduce the distortion themselves. This distortion can be treated in the prone position with or without the hip of the involved side flexed to approximately 30 degrees (Figs. 9.11 and 9.12).

Bullseye HTP

This extremely common HTP is frequently identified when patients present complaining of low back pain. Bullseye HTP tends to present over the anatomical region of the piriformis. The patient will press a thumb, knuckle, or fist deep into their buttock. Pain from this distortion may be associated with radicular pain extending to the foot.

In patients presenting with the complaint of "sciatica," it is important to treat this distortion before diagnosis is confirmed. Treatment of bullseye HTP can be performed with the patient in many different positions, including standing, prone, and prone with the hip flexed. In pregnancy, bullseye HTP can be treated with the patient on their side (Figs. 9.13 and 9.14).

Superior cluneal nerve HTP

There are branches of the superior cluneal nerve that travel over the iliac crest. Superior cluneal nerve HTPs are identified as tender areas along the iliac crest and are a common cause of low back pain. This

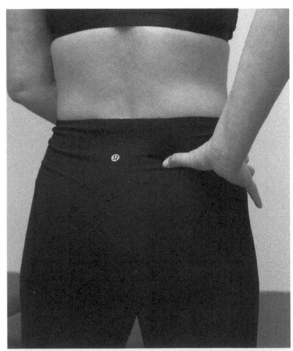

FIGURE 9.11
Posterior superior iliac spine (PSIS) herniated trigger point (HTP) patient gesture

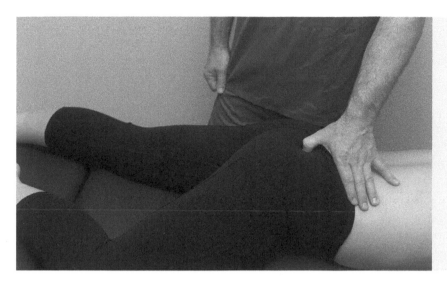

FIGURE 9.12
Posterior superior iliac spine (PSIS) herniated trigger point (HTP) treatment, prone

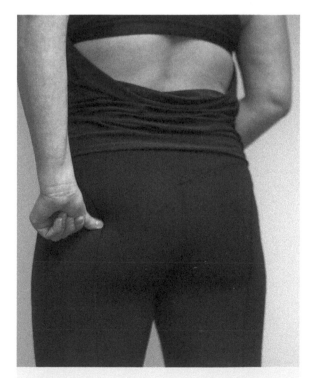

FIGURE 9.13
Bullseye herniated trigger point (HTP) patient gesture

may be the etiology of pain that wraps anteriorly into the groin. Injection of superior cluneal nerves that have been entrapped has been discussed in the literature. Reducing these HTPs can be very effective at relieving low back pain with or without radiculopathy. Treatment in the prone position or child's pose can be useful (Fig. 9.15).

Continuum distortions (CDs) of the lumbar region

CDs occur at any fascia–bone connection that a patient identifies. Common CDs in the lumbar region are found at the fascia–bone connections of the lumbar spinous process, PSIS, iliac crest, and sacrum (Fig. 9.16).

With spinous process CDs, the practitioner should be aware that distortions are often found on the lateral edges of the spinous process and not on the most posterior aspect of the spinous process. If a patient identifies a CD on a spinous process, ensure no serious trauma has occurred so that a fracture is not missed (Fig. 9.17).

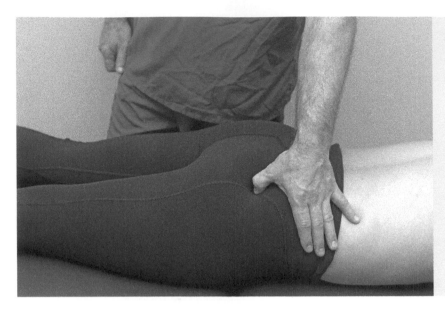

FIGURE 9.14
Bullseye herniated trigger point (HTP) treatment, prone

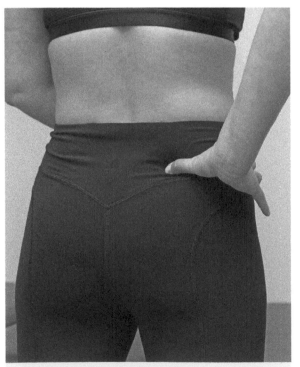

FIGURE 9.15
Superior cluneal nerve herniated trigger point (HTP)

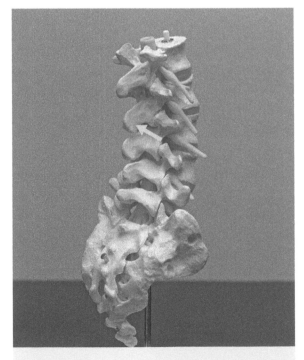

FIGURE 9.16
Common lumbar continuum distortion (CD) locations

Folding distortions (FDs) of the lumbar region

Lumbar refolding distortions (rFDs)

The patient gesture associated with folding of the spine is a holding of the spine. One hand may be placed flat on the spine (Fig. 9.18), or both hands can be placed over the lower back. The back of the hand resting over the lumbar spine, along with the verbal complaint of pain deep in the spine, is a common presentation for FDs of the lumbar spine. If a patient draws a line horizontally across the spine, this can represent an rFD (Fig. 9.19). Pain that improves or gets worse as the day goes on also provides a clue as to the type of FD present, if the history of injury does not provide the diagnosis (see below).

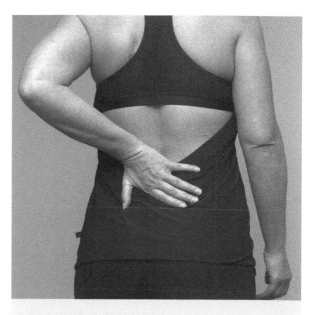

FIGURE 9.18
Lumbar folding patient gesture

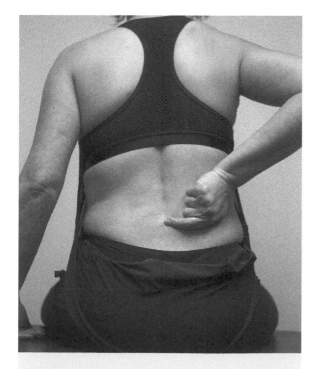

FIGURE 9.17
Lumbar continuum distortion (CD) patient gesture

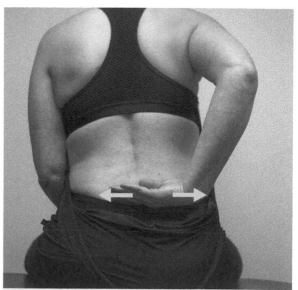

FIGURE 9.19
Lumbar refolding patient gesture

Unfolding distortions (uFDs) of the spine

Any mechanism of force that causes a spinal segment to unfold, torque, and incompletely refold is called an unfolding distortion (uFD). Patients with uFDs of the spine will often say that their pain is better in the morning, worsening as the day goes on. When treating an unfolding of the spine, the force vector applied to the spinal segment should separate the affected vertebrae, recreating the direction of the injury if it is known. Treatment should not be painful.

Lumbar uFDs are associated with relief upon traction of the affected segments: axial compression of the spine makes the pain worse. These patients often report significantly less pain after sleeping. When a person is lying horizontal in bed, the spinal segment no longer has the effect of gravity attempting to compress it and the spine naturally becomes longer. Each spinal segment is unfolding, providing the patient with relief. When a person stands up, gravity begins to compress the spine, and so patients with unfolding injuries complain of pain when standing.

Treatment of uFDs

Traditional manual medicine techniques are very effective at treating this distortion if unfolding the vertebral segment is incorporated into existing techniques. In the unfolding treatment, traction is applied to the joint or vertebra until the wrinkled fascia unfolds, often with an audible "pop".

Lumbar roll technique

The lumbar roll technique is traditionally used after a practitioner determines in which direction the affected lumbar segment is rotated. This is done by placing the hands behind the iliac crest while the patient is supine. When the hip is lifted straight up, one of the hips will often lift more easily, allowing the lumbar spine to rotate in the same direction that the lumbar spine is rotated (Fig. 9.20). With the lumbar roll, the practitioner then forces the vertebral segment in the other direction (Fig. 9.21). If the lumbar spine is rotated to the right, then the practitioner places the patient on the left side. With the FDM, another dimension of motion of the vertebral

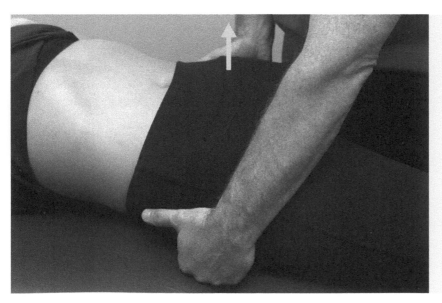

FIGURE 9.20
Motion testing for lumbar rotation

segments is added, either compression (refolding) or expansion (unfolding) of the vertebral complex. For the purpose of this discussion, the vertebral complex is defined as two vertebrae separated by a disc. Through verbal description and body language, the patient will identify the type of FD they are experiencing, i.e. if they patient wakes with little pain but notices pain when getting up and moving, they are likely to have an uFD; but if being upright during the day, compressing the spine through lifting, or carrying a pack, makes the pain worse, they likely have a uFD. The lumbar roll technique for an a uFD is performed with a traction force with the intent of gapping the two vertebrae (Fig. 9.22).

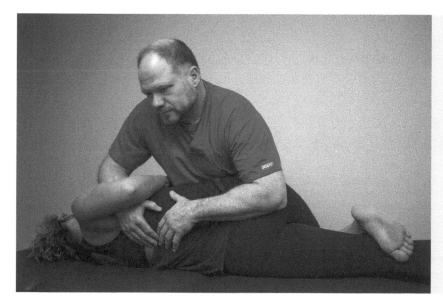

FIGURE 9.21
Lumbar roll set-up

FIGURE 9.22
Lumbar roll technique with
unfolding

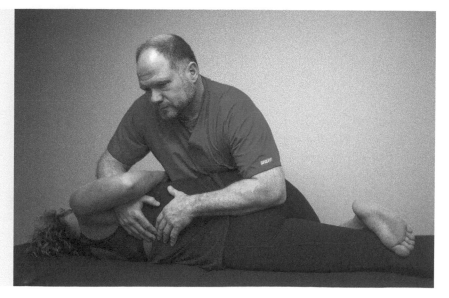

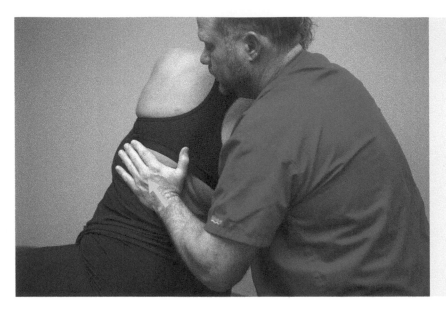

FIGURE 9.23
Chair technique with lumbar unfolding

Seated chair technique

In the seated chair technique, the patient is positioned straddling a chair with their arms on the back of the chair. (The treatment table can also be used instead of the chair, and in this case, the patient would straddle the table.) If a uFD has been identified by history or gesture, then the lumbar spine needs to be unfolded, separating the affected vertebrae. The patient is rotated to their more comfortable side , and an unfolding force is applied to the lumbar spine (Fig. 9.23).

Inversion table

Inversion therapy, which is discussed later (see Chapter 19), can be used to unfold the spine (Fig. 9.24). When a patient is on the inversion table, the vertebral segments are separated by the weight of the body and gravity. If this feels "right," then it is the right treatment. If traction or inversion does not feel good, then a refolding or another (painful) distortion is present. While on the inversion table, the patient can be rotated towards the position of comfort, allowing for further unfolding (Fig. 9.25).

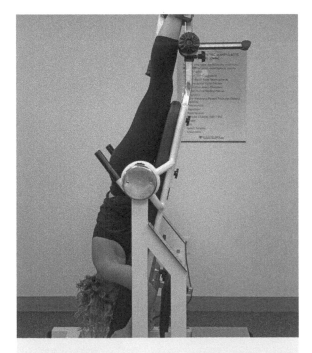

FIGURE 9.24
Inversion therapy for spinal unfolding

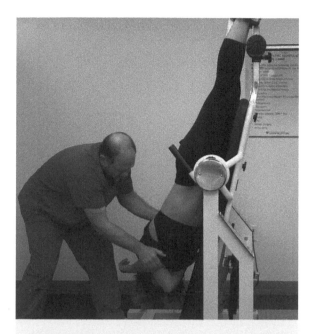

FIGURE 9.25
Inversion therapy for spinal unfolding with added rotation

Hallelujah technique

This technique can be used to effect an unfolding in the lumbar spine. When the patient's hands are placed over the lumbar spine, the practitioner can direct force into the lumbar region, causing a separation of the vertebrae. With the hands in different positions, this technique can also be used effectively on the thoracic spine (Fig. 9.26).

To apply the Hallelujah technique to the lumbar region, the patient is instructed to place their hands on their lower back. The practitioner places their hands through the patient's arms and holds them while the patient leans back into the practitioner. While the patient is supported by the provider, they sit down as the practitioner thrusts upward, maximizing the gapping of the low back. This technique is best used when the patient is equal in size or

smaller than the practitioner (Figs. 9.27 and 9.28). If the patient is larger than the provider can safely support, this technique can be modified with the patient seated (Fig. 9.29).

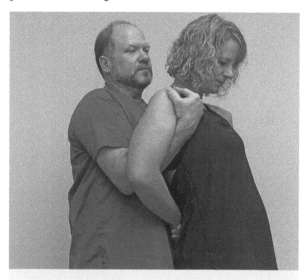

FIGURE 9.26
Hallelujah technique for lumbar unfolding treatment

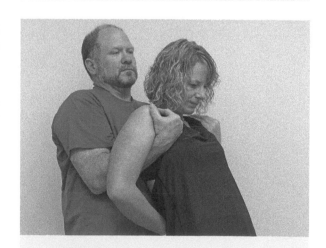

FIGURE 9.27
Hallelujah technique for lumbar unfolding: hand placement

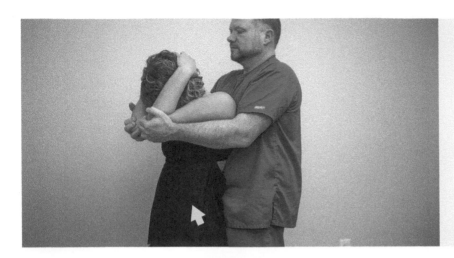

FIGURE 9.28
Hallelujah technique for lumbar unfolding: force vector

FIGURE 9.29A, B
Hallelujah technique for lumbar unfolding treatment, seated

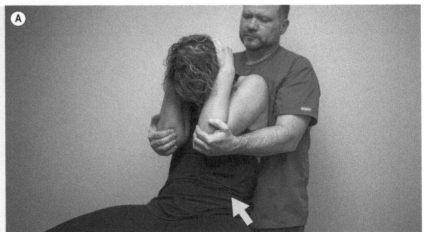

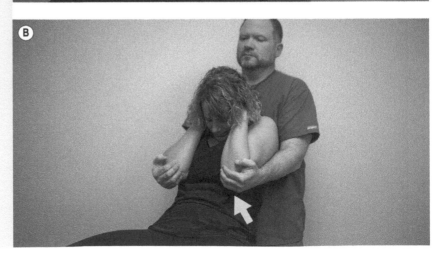

Lumbar rFDs

Patients with refolding of the lumbar region may demonstrate the distortion by cupping, squeezing, or holding the joint, followed by a sweeping or rubbing motion with a finger across the joint. These patients may attempt to find relief by bringing the joint under compression. Patients with rFDs of the spine will also indicate their pain is better in the evening, after a day of gravity compressing the spine, and worse in the morning, after their spine has decompressed during sleep. Pain in rFDs increases with traction, thus many patients with rFDs will not tolerate inversion therapy. When treating refolding injuries, compression is applied to the joint until the wrinkled folding fascia refolds, at which point it is released back to the neutral position, often with an audible click.

Treatment of rFDs of the spine

Lumbar roll

The lumbar roll technique is traditionally used after a practitioner determines which direction the affected lumbar segment is rotated (as described above and seen in Fig. 9.20). The practitioner then must force the vertebral segment in the other direction (Fig. 9.21). Through verbal description and gesture, the patient will identify the type of folding distortion they are experiencing. If a patient has less pain after being up on their feet or while carrying a backpack, the practitioner could infer that the lumbar roll should be performed with a compressive or refolding force (Fig. 9.30).

Seated chair technique

With the seated chair technique, the patient is positioned straddling the chair or treatment table as described above. When an rFD is identified in the low back, the patient is rotated and side bent towards the side of least pain. FDs are not painful to treat. When the rotational barrier is reached, and the patient is "locked out," a downward or compressive thrust is applied, refolding the lumbar complex (Fig. 9.31).

Axial compression

Simple compression (refolding) of the lumbar spine can be achieved by pressing straight down on a

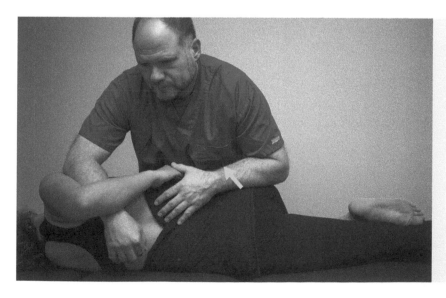

FIGURE 9.30
Lumbar roll technique with refolding

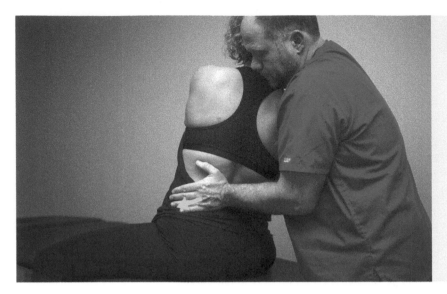

FIGURE 9.31
Chair technique with lumbar refolding

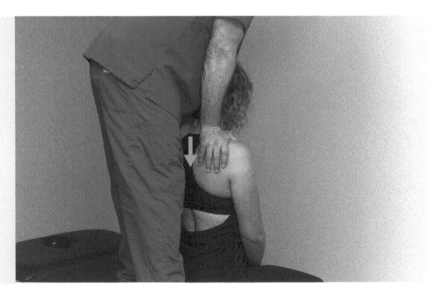

FIGURE 9.32
Lumbar refolding with axial compression

patient's shoulders while they are in the seated position (Fig. 9.29B). The patient sits on the treatment table with their feet on the floor. The practitioner stands behind the patient, placing their hands on the patient's shoulders. Before pressing down on the shoulders and compressing the spine, the trapezius and overlying tissue should be compressed and slid towards the cervical spine (Fig. 9.32), preventing traction being applied to the sides of the neck. A progressively increasing force is then applied, compressing the entire spine.

As each segment of the spine is compressed, subtle rotational movements may be required to achieve the level of compression needed to treat the rFD. The practitioner may accomplish this by turning the patient's torso to the point of ease and comfort while maintaining downward pressure, allowing the spine to compress further, and the next level in the spine to be addressed. The number and location of the segments being treated is assessed through practitioner palpation and feedback from the patient. Pain encountered in the spine during this treatment suggests that either the wrong rotational force is used at a segment, or a uFD is present. This uFD may need to be treated before additional refolding is performed.

If the force needed to compress the spine with the practitioner pressing down on the shoulders is not adequate, additional weight can be applied by the practitioner sitting on the shoulders of the patient. Care must be taken with this treatment: the relative size of practitioner and patient needs to be considered, as well as any health condition in the patient that contraindicate it, such as osteoporosis.

Relative contraindications for spinal refolding/compression

- Provider-patient size mismatch
- Rib pain or fractures
- Osteoporosis
- Feline body type
- Patient doesn't think compression would feel good
- Pain with test of compression (indicates the presence of an unfolding distortion.

Lumbar cylinder distortions (CyDs)

The gestures associated with cylinder distortions (CyDs) of the lumbar region are sweeping or squeezing of the low back. These complaints are often bizarre or unusual in presentation. Frequently, the cylinder complaint does not fit with the anatomical pathways of lumbar pain taught traditionally and pain may jump around, or even move up the back or spine. Patients may also be experiencing more intense pain than might be expected.

Treatment modalities for CyDs include the same manual and non-manual techniques described elsewhere. Cupping with movement and skin distraction with the plunger are favorites of many FDM practitioners. Favorite manual techniques include the double-thumb, squeegee, and skin rolling.

Lumbar tectonic fixations (TFs)

Tectonic fixations (TFs) are not associated with any patient gesture. The patient will describe their pain by indicating they feel stuck or like they need to "pop" and may seek relief through self-correction, where they articulate their lumbar spine by twisting and applying pressure in different ways. They may find significant relief with the application of heat. Heat is thought to thin the fluid in the fascia, making the tissues move more easily.

Lumbar roll

When a patient is complaining of the lumbar spine feeling like it is stuck or needs to pop, the lumbar roll technique can be used without additional unfolding or refolding forces being applied. The patient is assessed for lumbar rotation, as described above. If the patient is found to be rotated to the right, then the patient is placed on the left sided, and the lumbar spine is further rotated to the left. No gap or compression is emphasized during this treatment (Fig. 9.33).

Hallelujah technique

The Hallelujah technique described above for lumbar unfolding is also useful for lumbar TF. The execution of the Hallelujah for a lumbar TF is virtually identical for that of a lumbar uFD. The patient is instructed to

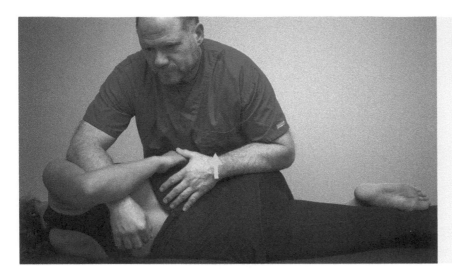

FIGURE 9.33
Lumbar roll technique for tectonic fixation (TF)

FIGURE 9.34
Chair technique for tectonic fixation (TF)

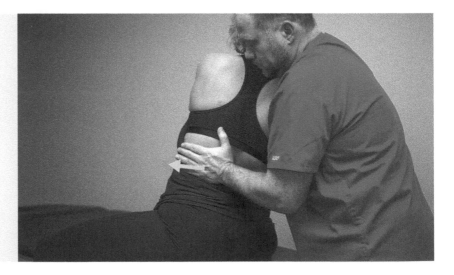

place their hands palm-out on their low back while, the practitioner directs force into the lumbar region, causing movement of the vertebrae. The practitioner places their hands through the patient's arms and holds them while the patient leans back into the patient. When the patient is supported by the provider, the patient then sits down as the provider thrusts upward, maximizing the gapping of the low back.

Seated chair technique

With the seated chair technique, the patient is positioned straddling the chair or treatment table. The patient is then rotated in one direction, while the thrust is applied in the opposite direction. In tectonic treatment, no compressing or separating vector is added to the force of the thrust (Fig. 9.34).

Often this region is divided into two separate conversations, but the division is frequently unclear when one considers the ubiquitous and seamless fascial network in the region. The complexity of the pelvic and sacral anatomy – with overlapping musculature, as well as a complex layering of the pelvic and sacral ligaments and tendons – provides nearly limitless locations for the development of fascial distortions. Even with a wide distribution of potential distortions, recurrent distortions in predictable locations have been identified.

Pelvic and sacral triggerbands

The incredibly complex intertwining of the fascial layers and matrix in this area make the possible location of triggerbands nearly endless: every muscle, ligament, and tendon has a fascial covering where triggerbands can form. The superficial fascial matrix of the pelvic region is also a common source of triggerbands. Triggerbands in this region, as in any region of the body, occur exactly where the patient demonstrates them and some frequently reccurring triggerbands have been named.

Inguinal triggerband

This triggerband usually begins near the pubic rami and travels laterally along the inguinal crease to the anterior superior iliac spine (ASIS). In other models these complaints are frequently diagnosed as round ligament pain, with fewer treatment options compared to the triggerband (Fig. 10.1).

Sacroiliac (SI) triggerband

Patients may identify lines of pain and tightness that closely correlate with the SI joint. These triggerbands may form at the tip of the coccyx and travel along the SI joint (Fig. 10.2).

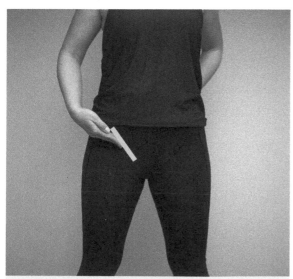

FIGURE 10.1
Inguinal triggerband

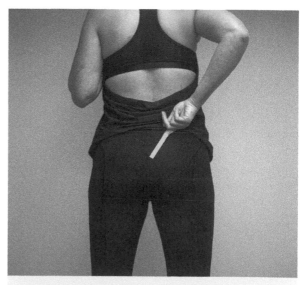

FIGURE 10.2
Sacroiliac (SI) triggerband

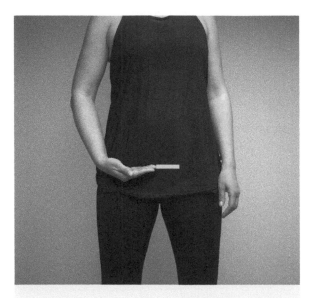

FIGURE 10.3
Pubic triggerband

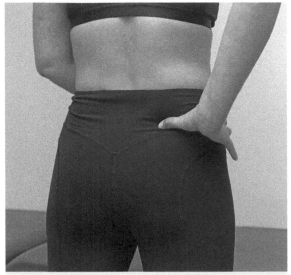

FIGURE 10.4
Superior cluneal nerve herniated trigger point (HTP)

Pubic triggerband

A linear band of pain across the region of the pubic symphysis described by the patient as "tight pulling" indicates a pubic triggerband (Fig. 10.3).

Pelvic and sacral herniated triggerpoints (HTPs)

Herniated triggerpoints (HTPs) in the pelvic/sacral region are identified with the same gesture and verbal description as any other region of the body: multiple fingers, a thumb, or knuckle pushing into a soft tissue area that is painful to palpation. Reduction of HTPs in the pelvic and sacral region is achieved using the same techniques as in other areas of the body.

Superior cluneal nerve HTP

Patients experiencing pelvic or low back pain may present with pain along the iliac crest. Branches of the superior cluneal nerve are associated with the iliac crest and each presents a potential avenue for the herniation of underlying fascial tissue (Fig. 10.4).

Medial cluneal nerve HTP

Patients may experience pain along the lateral edge of the sacrum. The patient pressing into the soft tissue near the lateral border of the sacrum with multiple fingers indicates a medial cluneal nerve HTP (Fig. 10.5).

Inferior cluneal nerve HTP

Patients complaining of pelvic pain may present with fingers pressing deep into the buttock at the area of the ischial tuberosity. This may also be referred to as a high hamstring strain. Multiple fingers pressing deep below the buttock is indicative of an inferior cluneal nerve HTP (Fig. 10.6).

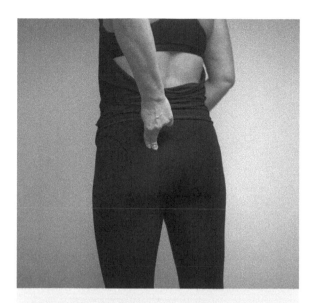

FIGURE 10.5
Medial cluneal nerve herniated trigger point (HTP)

Bullseye HTP

The area of the piriformis is a frequent source of pain in patients with pelvic, sacral, and even lumbar pain. This common distortion is identified with a knuckle, thumb, or multiple fingers pressing into the buttock (Fig. 10.7).

Posterior superior iliac spine (PSIS) HTP

A lipoma is commonly found a the posterior superior iliac spine (PSIS), and. patients may gesture to this area as a source of pain. Often the lipoma is not the etiology of pain but instead it is due to an HTP that is located deep in the lipoma. The practitioner can work around the lipoma to reduce the HTP. Generally, lipomas are more mobile and more solid feeling than HTPs (Fig. 10.8).

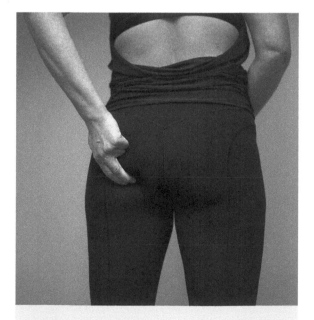

FIGURE 10.6
Inferior cluneal nerve herniated trigger point (HTP)

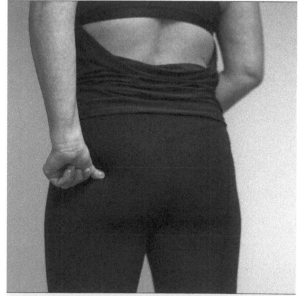

FIGURE 10.7
Bullseye herniated trigger point (HTP)

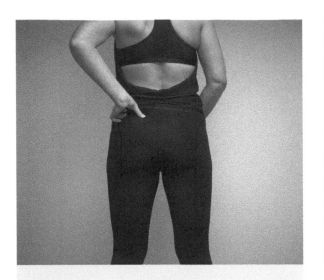

FIGURE 10.8
Posterior superior iliac spine (PSIS) herniated trigger point (HTP)

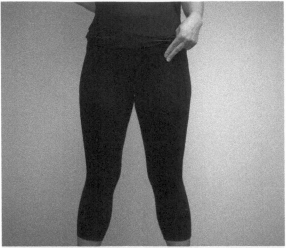

FIGURE 10.9
Anterior superior iliac spine (ASIS) herniated trigger point (HTP)

ASIS HTP

Patients have identified HTPs that are slightly medial or slightly lateral to the ASIS. The gesture remains the same as for any other HTP: multiple fingers, a thumb, or knuckle pressing into a soft tissue spot. This distortion is frequently seen in pregnant women (Fig. 10.9).

Inguinal/femoral HTP

This HTP is found in the inguinal region and may be associated with the femoral vessels (Fig. 10.10). Reduction of can be exceptionally painful. Various treatment strategies can be used to make reduction more efficient and less painful.

If a patient identifies an HTP in the groin region, the femoral artery and vessels should be carefully palpated – aggressive pressure in this area is not

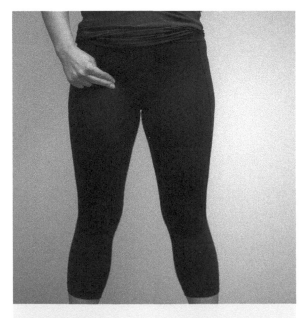

FIGURE 10.10
Inguinal herniated trigger point (HTP)

recommended. Once the distortion is identified, the patient can be placed supine. The patient then places both hands on their abdomen and lifts cephalad, pulling the abdomen and its contents up and away from the inguinal region (Fig. 10.11). This creates a vacuum-like force assisting with the reduction of the HTP by pulling the tissue back up into the abdomen.

External rotation of the hip while pressure is placed on the HTP can also help in the reduction of this HTP (Fig. 10.12A). With the practitioner's treating thumb on the HTP while applying pressure in the generally cephalad direction, the hip can be moved through external rotation and extension. This hip mobilization combined with the pressure of the thumb is often effective at reducing the HTP (Fig. 10.12B).

Pubic HTP

A patient may identify a pubic HTP by pressing multiple fingers into the soft tissue overlying the pubic region.

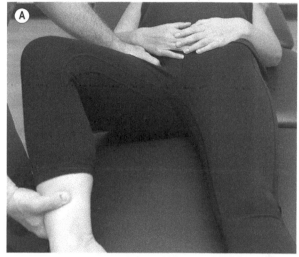

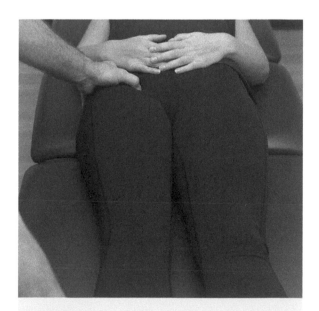

FIGURE 10.11
Inguinal herniated trigger point (HTP) treatment with patient assist

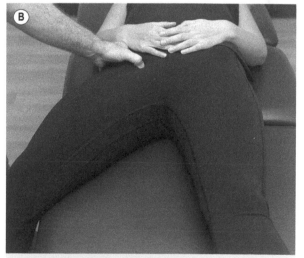

FIGURE 10.12A,B
Inguinal herniated trigger point (HTP) treatment with external hip rotation

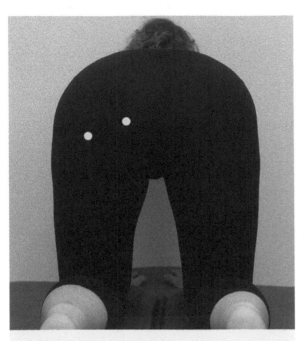

FIGURE 10.13
Common locations of pelvic floor herniated trigger points (HTPs)

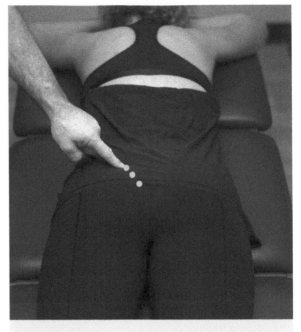

FIGURE 10.14
Sacral edge continuum distortions (CDs)

Pelvic floor HTP

Multiple fingers pressing into a painful area of the pelvic floor indicates a pelvic floor HTP. Positioning and directing pressure appropriately can be difficult when treating these distortions and this area of the body is sometimes difficult for people to discuss (Fig. 10.13).

Pelvis and sacrum continuum distortions (CDs)

Due to the extensive fascial coverings of the pelvis and sacrum, continuum distortions (CDs) may arise in many locations. As with all CD treatments, localization of the distortion is important to the effective and efficient reduction of the CD.

Sacral edge CDs

CDs along the lateral edge of the sacrum can be associated with pelvic and sacral pain as well as pain referred down into the lower extremity (Fig. 10.14).

PSIS CDs

CDs near the PSIS are due to the large amount of fascial tissue from the lower extremity musculature that attaches to the PSIS (Fig. 10.15).

Iliac crest CDs

Tender areas along the iliac crest identified as single spots of pain are found in patients with pelvic and sacral pain as well as low back pain.

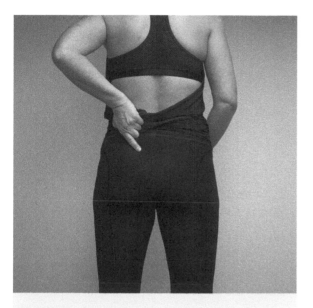

FIGURE 10.15
Posterior superior iliac spine (PSIS) continuum distortions (CDs)

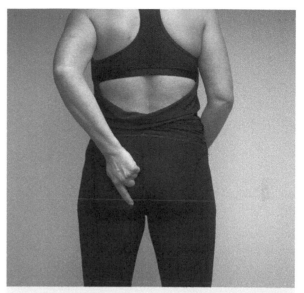

FIGURE 10.16
Ischial tuberosity continuum distortions (CDs)

Ischial tuberosity CDs

Single spots of tenderness identified along the ischial tuberosity indicate CDs. This is a difficult location to treat since the bony edge where the CDs often form is very narrow and requires excellent technique to localize the distortion on the tuberosity (Fig. 10.16).

Coccyx CDs

CDs associated with the coccyx need to be treated with very focused technique and minimal force to effectively treat this distortion and relieve pain (Fig. 10.17).

Pubic symphysis CDs

The symphysis pubis has a fascia–bone continuum that, when distorted, can cause malalignment

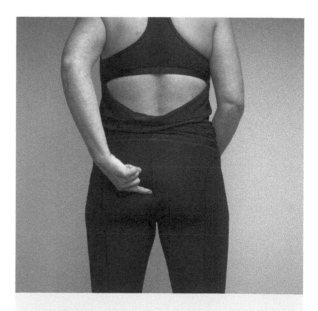

FIGURE 10.17
Coccyx continuum distortions (CDs)

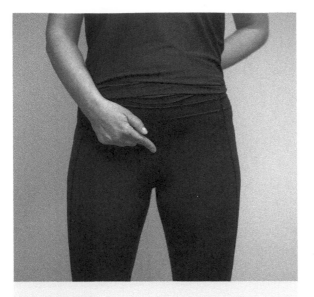

FIGURE 10.18
Pubic symphysis continuum distortions (CDs)

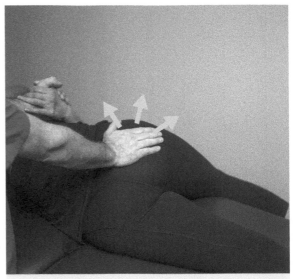

FIGURE 10.19
Scissors technique for inverted continuum distortions (CDs)

of the symphysis. Correction of CDs identified in this area can rapidly correct pubic symphysis pain (Fig. 10.18).

Inverted CDs

Inverted CDs are found on the dorsal aspect of the sacrum. Traditional everted CD treatment techniques can be used to address inverted CDs. Thrust techniques can also be used to pull the stuck or inverted fascial fibers from the bone.

Scissors technique

The scissors technique is an example of a thrust technique useful for addressing inverted CDs. In this technique, the patient lies on the opposite side to the inverted sacral CD, then extends their leg on the side of the CD until it hangs off the table. The practitioner stands behind the patient and grasps the

patient's hand on the side they are lying on, then uses the patient's arm to rotate the patient until a barrier to rotation is reached. Keeping the patient's arm near their waist helps lock the rotational force into the sacrum. The practitioner then places the thenar eminence of their other hand on the lateral margin of the sacrum, and applies thrust to the sacrum, pulling fascial fibers from the sacral base (Fig. 10.19). Multiple vectors of force can be used in this treatment.

SI folding distortions (FDs)

Folding distortions (FDs) of the SI joint are identified by a patient cupping or holding the SI joint (Fig. 10.20).

Scissors technique

The scissors technique can also be used to treat sacral folding. Generally, if a patient is placed on their side

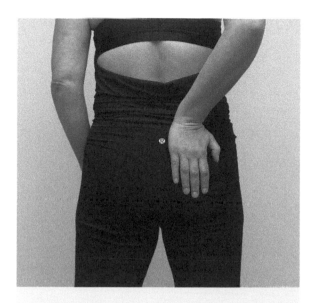

FIGURE 10.20

Sacroiliac (SI) folding distortions (FDs)

for this technique and the thenar eminence of the practitioner is placed on the side they are not lying on, then the lateral edge engaged by the thenar eminence can be thought to be refolding, and the lower SI joint to be unfolding. Since unfolding treatments should not hurt, if the scissors treatment is painful, then the patient should be placed on the opposite side, and the treatment attempted again (Fig. 10.21).

Sacral high-velocity, low-amplitude (HVLA) technique

HVLA can be used to treat FDs of the sacrum. In this technique, the patient is placed on their side, and the forearm of the practitioner is used to thrust and refold the sacrum (Fig. 10.22).

Frog-leg hip technique

The frog-leg technique used for the hip can also be used to treat FDs of the SI joint. The practitioner

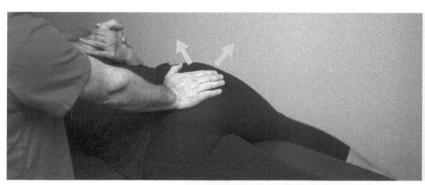

FIGURE 10.21

Scissors technique for sacroiliac (SI) folding distortions (FDs)

FIGURE 10.22

Sacral high-velocity, low-amplitude (HVLA) for folding distortions (FDs)

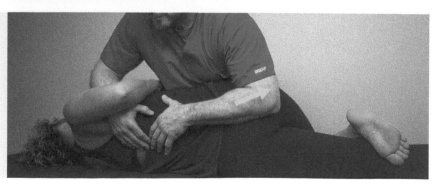

grasps the ankle on the side to be treated, while the other is placed on the ipsilateral knee. With the hip flexed to 90 degrees, the knee is placed under maximum flexion, and the foot is then rotated around the femur and hip joint, placing a rotational force into the hip joint. When the hip is rotated internally, the SI joint can be thought to be unfolding (Fig. 10.23).

Pubic symphysis FD

FDs of the pubic symphysis often present with patients describing pain deep in the pubic symphysis, accompanied by a gesture of holding the pubic symphysis (Fig. 10.24). This distortion can be treated with pubic unfolding. To treat this condition, the patient is placed supine with knees bent and their feet resting on the table. Muscle energy techniques

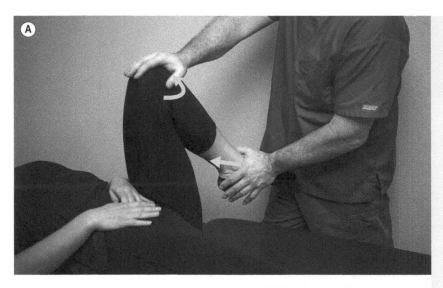

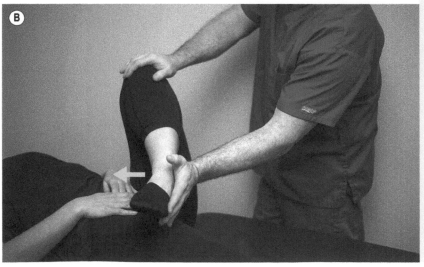

FIGURE 10.23A, B
Frog-leg technique for sacroiliac (SI) folding distortions (FDs)

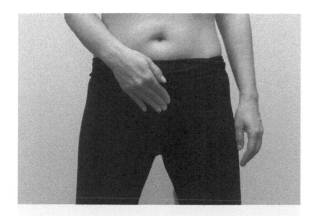

FIGURE 10.24
Pubic symphysis folding distortion (FD)

or a thrust mechanism can be used to separate the knees, unfolding the pubic symphysis. As a folding treatment, this technique should not be painful. If the patient identifies pretreatment pain, then an unfolding is not present, and a different diagnosis should be considered (Fig. 10.25).

Leg tug

Unfolding the SI joint can be performed with a patient lying prone. The ankle on the side of the SI joint to be unfolded is grasped, and traction is applied. The leg is then maneuvered to create a gapping feeling in the hip and SI joint on the side being treated. If this is not painful, a thrust can be applied, gapping the hip and sacrum (Fig. 10.26).

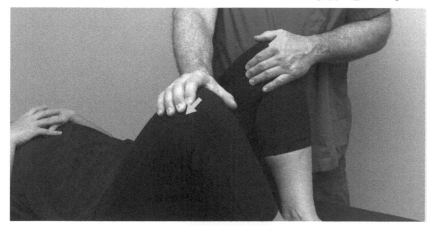

FIGURE 10.25
Pubic symphysis unfolding distortion (uFD) treatment

FIGURE 10.26
Sacroiliac (SI) joint unfolding distortion (uFD) treatment: leg tug

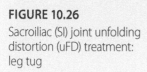

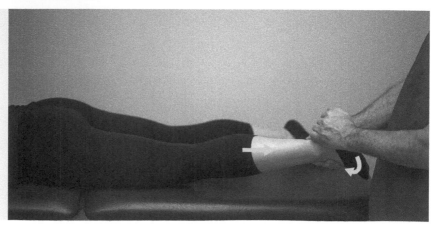

Pelvis and sacrum cylinder distortions (CyDs)

Cylinders in the pelvic and sacral region may be associated with bizarre and unusual pain presentations. Cylinder distortions (CyDs) in this area may be responsible for some complaints associated with chronic pelvic pain. Body language associated with cylinders in this area include sweeping or squeezing (Fig. 10.27).

Sacrum cupping

If the patient gesture is a sweeping or squeezing over the sacrum, cupping can be effectively used to treat this cylinder distortion. The cup is placed over the location of the identified CyD, and the patient is then encouraged to move. Movement should include flexion, extension, twisting, side bending, and walking (Fig. 10.28).

Pelvic skin rolling and double-thumb techniques

In other areas of the sacrum and pelvis where a cup may not be applied, double-thumb technique

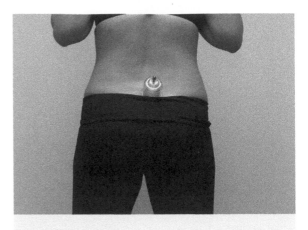

FIGURE 10.28
Sacral region cupping

and skin rolling can be used to lift the skin, allowing the tangled coils of superficial fascia to uncoil.

Pelvis and sacrum tectonic fixations (TFs)

Tectonic fixations (TFs) of the pelvis and sacral area include TF of the hip and SI joint. If a TF of either of these joints occurs, applying heat to the joint before treatment is appropriate. After heating the joint, a slow rhythmic pumping of the joint can be performed to mobilize the joint fluid. Once the pump has been performed, any of the thrust maneuvers can be applied to separate the tectonically-fixed fascial layers.

Frog-leg hip technique

The frog-leg hip technique can be used to mobilize fluid in the hip and SI joints. A thrust added to the frog-leg technique can be used to treat TFs of both the SI joint and the hip joint.

Scissors technique

The scissors technique can be used following a pump technique to mobilize a tectonic SI joint.

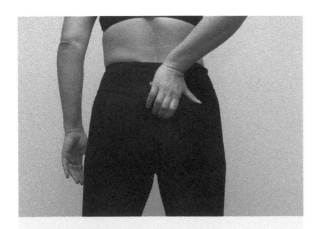

FIGURE 10.27
Sacral region cylinder distortion (CyD)

The complaint of shoulder pain is widespread. It is essential for the practitioner to routinely perform a proper evaluation so that abnormalities can be quickly identified. Consistency in the shoulder examination will allow the practitioner to compare a patient's range of movement (ROM) to the normal range in other patients. It is also helpful to compare one shoulder to the other in the same patient in order to evaluate the differences in ROM, rhythm, and speed of movement.

One frequently-used pattern of evaluation is as follows: the patient extends their arms straight out in front of them (Fig. 11.1A) then moves their arms to the side (Fig. 11.1B). They then abduct their shoulders, ending with their hands up over their head, with elbows fully extended (Fig. 11.1C). External rotation of the shoulder can be evaluated with the hands placed behind the head, and the elbows pushed back (Fig. 11.1D). Internal rotation is measured by placing the back of the patient's hand flat on the spine

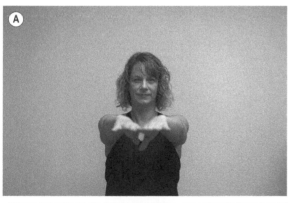
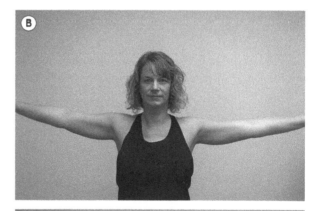
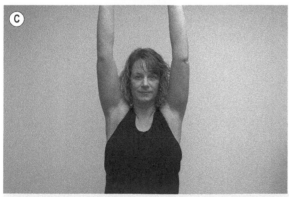
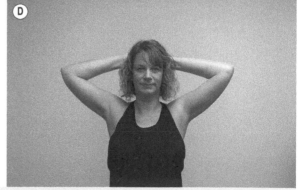

FIGURE 11.1A–D
Shoulder examination

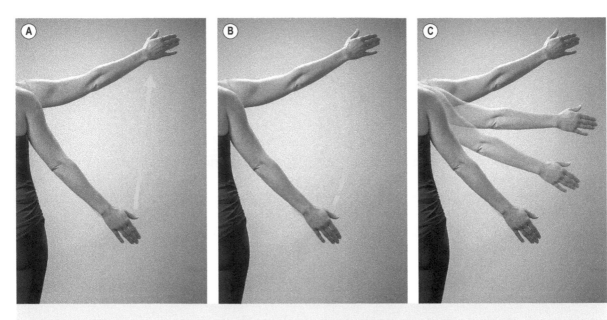

FIGURE 11.2A–C
Assessing the speed and smoothness of shoulder movement

and then raising the hand as far up the spine towards the head as possible. This movement should be symmetrical on both sides.

When observing a patient perform shoulder ROM, it is important to keep in mind the speed (Fig. 11.2A, B) at which the arm moves, and if there is stepping (Fig. 11.2C) or catching with the movement. The height that the hand can be raised above the waist should be be monitored and compared (Fig. 11.3). The amount of flaring of the elbow from the trunk (Fig. 11.4) is also a good indicator of function, and the distance from the body to the elbow should be symmetrical. When evaluating a patient's internal rotation of the shoulder, the practitioner should monitor hand direction and which way the fingers are pointing (Fig. 11.5), as well as whether the patient's hand can rotate when the palm is placed flat on their back (Fig. 11.6).

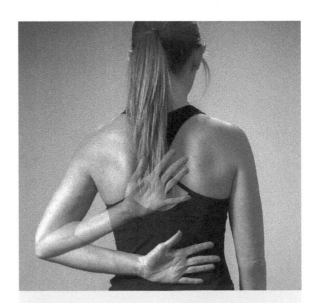

FIGURE 11.3
Internal rotation of shoulder

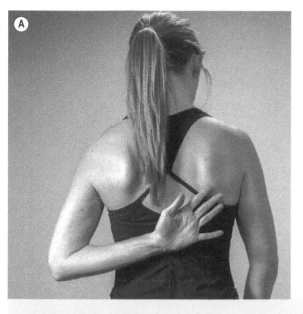

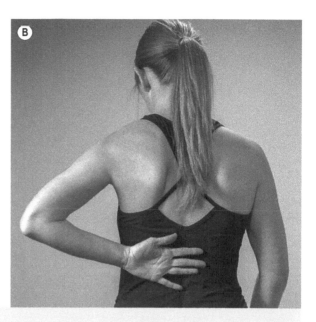

FIGURE 11.4A, B
Observing the distance from elbow to body

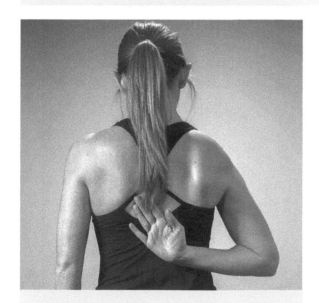

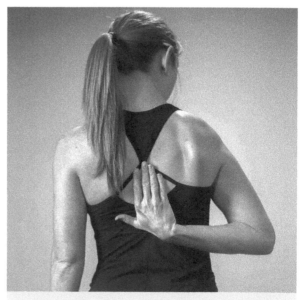

FIGURE 11.5
The practitioner should take note of the direction
the fingers and hand are pointing

FIGURE 11.6
Hand rotation

Shoulder triggerbands

There are triggerbands found in the shoulder region that are so prevalent they have been named (Fig. 11.7). These are classic pathways that patients routinely identify. It is helpful to have a working knowledge of the typical origins and terminations of these common triggerbands so that the practitioner can ensure that the whole triggerband is treated. Often a patient may only demonstrate a small portion of the triggerband pathway, but treating the entire pathway ensures the entire distortion is treated, closing the triggerband completely.

Star triggerband

The so-called star triggerband was designated the "star of the show" by Dr Typaldos as it was the first triggerband treated (Fig. 11.8). This triggerband is located along the thoracic spine, generally beginning near the level of T6, running superior and parallel to

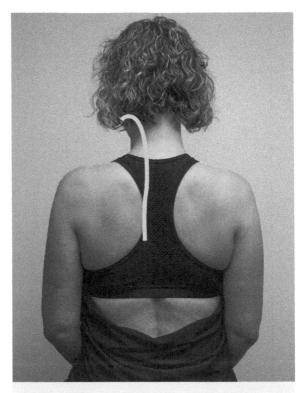

FIGURE 11.8
Star triggerband

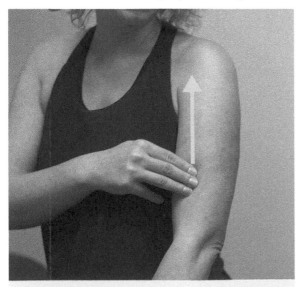

FIGURE 11.7
Gesture indicating presence and location of a shoulder triggerband

the spine, and overlying the paraspinal muscles. The star triggerband continues to transition into the neck region and passes along the occiput, usually ending at the mastoid, although variations in which the triggerband continues up over the scalp are frequently reported. The distance of the triggerband from the spinous process is also variable, and it is essential to obtain patient feedback to ensure that the practitioner is treating the triggerband. The patient should be experiencing tenderness along the entire pathway of the triggerband. It is important to remember that while the star triggerband may be associated with the paraspinal muscles, it commonly occurs in the superficial fascial layers. This fascial matrix is where many distortions occur.

Sometimes it is difficult to get traditionally trained manual therapists to understand that the superficial fascial matrix is where these distortions exist, and that they are not necessarily muscular in origin. The potentially shallow nature of the triggerband is important to consider, as this changes the angle and depth required for treatment. The goal of each triggerband treatment is to untwist the twisted fascial fibers in order to re-approximate the fascial myofibroblasts. If the practitioner can provide just enough force and depth to achieve that re-approximation, treatment will be less uncomfortable and much better tolerated by the patient. While triggerband treatment is painful, pain is not the goal of treatment.

Anterior shoulder triggerband

This triggerband is commonly demonstrated by patients experiencing both shoulder and cervical pain. It is generally located near the elbow and runs up the arm, anterior to the intermuscular septum, and over the biceps, typically continuing slightly anterior of the tip of the shoulder, across the upper trapezius region before finishing on the ipsilateral mastoid. Treatment of this entire triggerband can be performed even when only a small portion is demonstrated. Closing the entire triggerband will prevent it from reforming (Fig. 11.9). As with all triggerbands, it is important not to get distracted by the muscular anatomy. In this case, the anterior shoulder triggerband may have no association with the underlying anatomy of the biceps muscle.

Posterior shoulder triggerband

The posterior shoulder triggerband starts below the elbow and extends superiorly towards the shoulder, along the posterior aspect of the arm overlying the triceps region and commonly passing posterior to the tip of the shoulder. It then travels along the upper trapezius region, crosses midline at the spinal level of

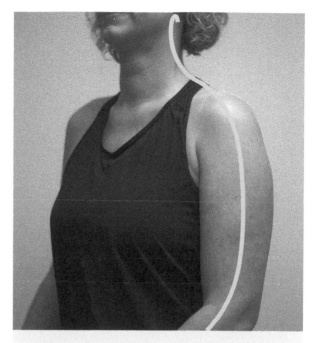

FIGURE 11.9
Anterior shoulder triggerband

C7-T1, and finally ends at the contralateral mastoid process (Fig. 11.10).

Shoulder–mastoid triggerband

The shoulder–mastoid triggerband is another distortion often displayed by patients complaining of both shoulder and neck pain. It is located near the tip of the shoulder and extends to the ipsilateral mastoid. During treatment, the practitioner may identify a supraclavicular herniated trigger point (HTP) along the course. Treating this relatively short triggerband can have powerful therapeutic implications (Fig. 11.11).

Scapular triggerband

Two separate locations are often referred to as the scapular triggerband. One follows the scapular ridge, while the other travels in a U-shape, approximating

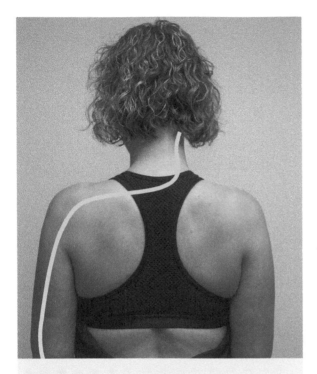

FIGURE 11.10
Posterior shoulder triggerband

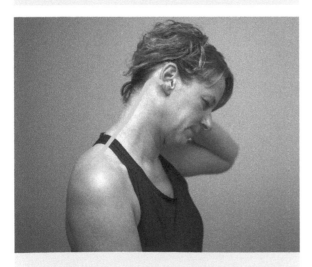

FIGURE 11.11
Shoulder–mastoid triggerband

the edge of the scapula. Both may be identified by a patient gesture. Patients with a U-shaped scapular triggerband may rely more on a verbal description of tightness and pulling, because this region is difficult for some patients to reach and provide the appropriate gesture (Fig. 11.12).

Shoulder herniated triggerpoints (HTPs)

HTPs of the shoulder region are a common distortion identified by patients presenting with complaints of shoulder pain. Often these distortions are associated with a limitation in ROM, pain, and aching (often worse at night). Remember that the HTP is thought to be associated with the superficial

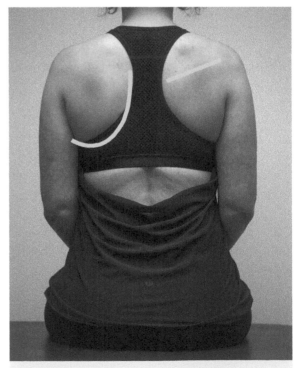

FIGURE 11.12
Triggerbands commonly seen on the scapula

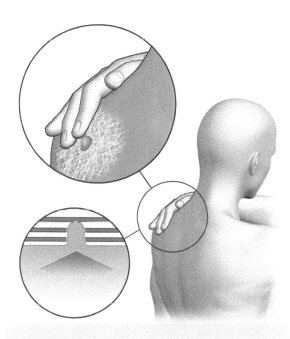

FIGURE 11.13
Herniated trigger point (HTP) traveling along nerve

cutaneous nerves which pass through the matrix of the superficial fascia. This penetration through the matrix may serve as a weak spot, allowing for the herniation of tissue up along the nerve (Fig. 11.13). The mechanism helps explain the pain associated with both having and reducing HTPs. Treatment of HTPs commonly causes bruising, possibly related to the fact that vessels accompany the nerve through the matrix as a neurovascular bundle (nerve, artery, and vein) and reduction of the HTP may disrupt some of the branches of the vascular supply. The association of HTPs with the superficial cutaneous nerves also provides a convenient nomenclature for HTPs.

Supraclavicular HTP (SCHTP)

Supraclavicular HTP (SCHTP) is one of the most frequently encountered HTPs in patients complaining of either cervical or shoulder pain. The SCHTP is considered to be the number one distortion responsible for the loss of cervical rotation, shoulder abduction, and internal rotation.

There are two variations of the SCHTP. The more common posterior SCHTP is found posterior to the line connecting the mastoid and the tip of the shoulder (Fig. 11.14). The anterior SCHTP is found anterior to the line connecting the shoulder and mastoid. Both HTPs can be exquisitely tender to treat, so caution and appropriate technique are advised (Fig. 11.15).

Deltoid HTP

The deltoid HTP is found at the neurovascular bundle associated with the deltoid insertion. This point is often described by patients with multiple fingers kneading the soft tissue of this area of the deltoid insertion and between the biceps and triceps. This distortion may be found and treated in patients with decreased internal rotation, even with the absence of gesture (Fig. 11.16).

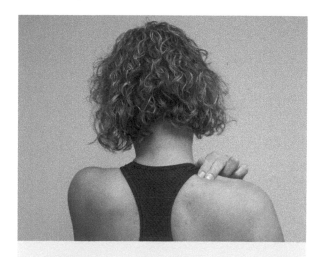

FIGURE 11.14
Posterior supraclavicular herniated trigger point (SCHTP)

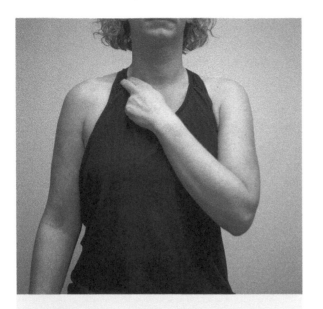

FIGURE 11.15
Anterior supraclavicular herniated trigger point (SCHTP)

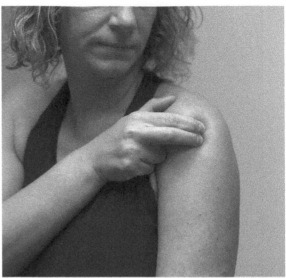

FIGURE 11.17
Subacromial herniated trigger point (HTP)

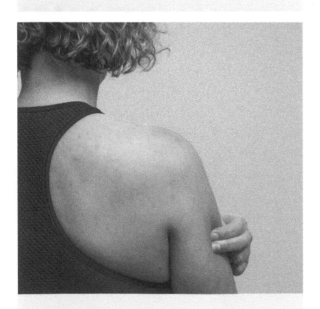

FIGURE 11.16
Patient gesture indicating presence and location of a deltoid herniated trigger point (HTP)

Subacromial HTP

The subacromial HTP is found underneath the acromion of the shoulder (Fig. 11.17) and is often identified as the source of pain for shoulder abduction. It may be found only in a small portion of the subacromial space, or it may be associated with the entire space. This distortion is routinely associated with the orthopedic diagnosis of impingement syndrome: the HTP itself may be what is being impinged during abduction of the shoulder. Reduction of subacromial HTP may be best achieved with the patient lying on the opposite shoulder. Traction of the arm can be applied to gap the subacromial space and ease reduction of the HTP (Fig. 11.18).

Subscapular HTP

The subscapular HTP is identified when the patient presses multiple fingers into the area of the subscapular neurovascular bundle on the posterior shoulder. Reduction of this HTP can be difficult, and the

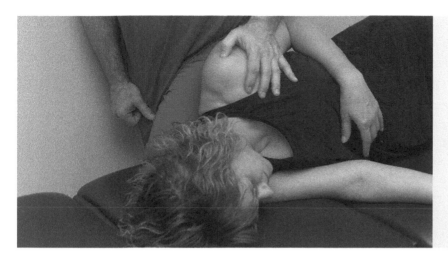

FIGURE 11.18
Patient placement for treatment of subacromial herniated trigger point (HTP)

appropriate vector should be identified before attempting a reduction. The vector is determined by locating the most painful direction on palpation (Fig. 11.19).

Suprascapular HTP

This HTP is identified when the patient reaches over the top of the shoulder and presses multiple fingers into the posterior aspect of their shoulder (Fig. 11.20).

Pectoral HTP

The pectoral HTP is found in the upper chest when the patient gestures with multiple fingers into the soft tissue of the pectoral region (Fig. 11.21).

Scapulothoracic HTP

Pain in the region of the scapulothoracic joint is a common complaint (Fig. 11.22) and is very often associated with shoulder, cervical, and thoracic pain. When treating this distortion, it is important to position the arm to create scapular winging as this will prevent the reduction force applied to the HTP from aggravating the scapulothoracic cartilage (Fig. 11.23A). Using the treatment table to create

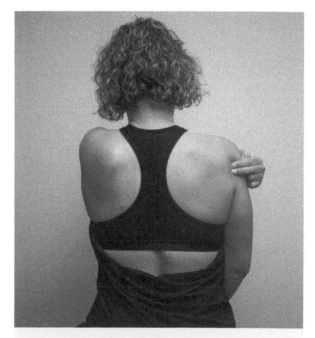

FIGURE 11.19
Subscapular herniated trigger point (HTP)

flexion of the thoracic spine can assist in the reduction of this HTP (Fig. 11.23B), or alternatively, the patient can accentuate thoracic flexion by hunching over a peanut ball.

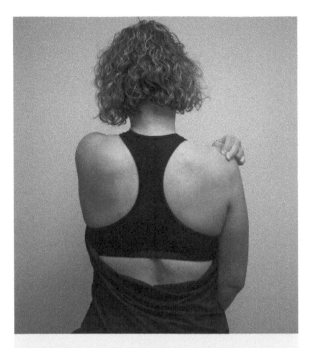

FIGURE 11.20
Suprascapular herniated trigger point (HTP)

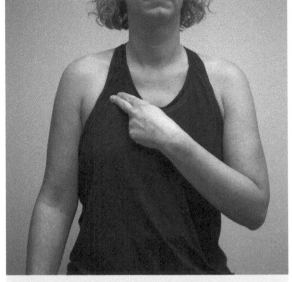

FIGURE 11.21
Pectoral herniated trigger point (HTP)

Shoulder continuum distortions (CDs)

Continuum distortions (CDs) occur wherever the patient identifies them. The gesture is a single finger pointing at a single spot of pain. Since the entire bony surface is covered in fascia, any bony surface can have a CD, but as with other distortions in the shoulder, there are some areas where CDs commonly occur. When treating CDs, the patient's gesture is critical when identifying the specific spot to treat. If a patient is experiencing a loss of ROM in one plane, then the practitioner should look for the CD causing the restriction, even in the absence of appropriate gesture.

Scapulothoracic CDs

The fascia–bone continuum in the scapulothoracic area is frequently subjected to stresses sufficient to

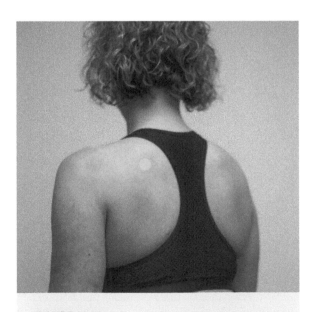

FIGURE 11.22
Scapulothoracic herniated trigger point (HTP)

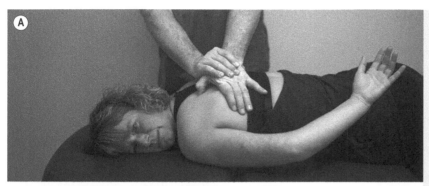

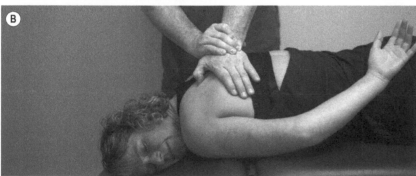

FIGURE 11.23A, B
Patient positioning for treatment of scapulothoracic herniated trigger point (HTP)

cause a CD. As with HTPs in this region, it is important to recognize that the tissue around this joint can become erythematous with persistent treatment (Fig. 11.24).

Glenohumeral CDs

CDs can occur along the glenohumeral region of the shoulder. The patient's gesture will guide the practitioner to the precise location.

Clavicular CDs

The clavicle may have CDs at the sternal junction as well as the acromial end.

Acromial CDs

This CD is often found when patients complain of shoulder pain. While all CDs are tender to treat, this particular CD is located in a sensitive area of the

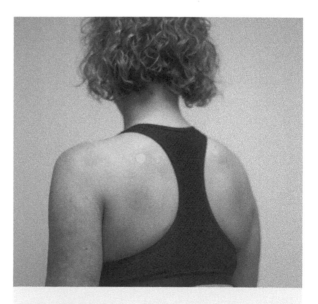

FIGURE 11.24
Scapulothoracic continuum distortion (CD)

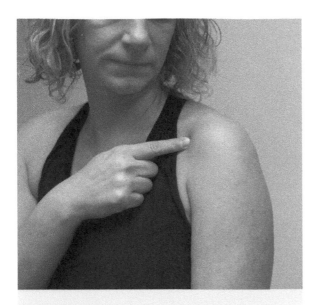

FIGURE 11.25
Acromial continuum distortion (CD)

shoulder, so caution and precise focus of force are recommended when treating it (Fig. 11.25).

Shoulder folding distortions (FDs)

The shoulder joint is surrounded by a fascial matrix that expands and collapses and is designed to absorb force. Compression of the matrix is referred to as refolding, and expansion of the matrix is called unfolding. If the fascial matrix can refold when forces are applied in one direction, it makes sense that it would unfold when forces are applied in the opposite direction, therefore the fascia of the shoulder can unfold and refold in many different directions and planes.

The gesture associated with FDs can be subtle. The patient will describe their pain by holding the joint. A hand placed over their shoulder, accompanied by a complaint of pain deep inside the joint, is one of the classic descriptions of a shoulder FD

(Fig. 11.26). The shoulder may feel unstable to the patient, but examination does not demonstrate any objective shoulder instability. Dr Typaldos identified the patient's interpretation or "sense" of instability as an FD. If a joint was unstable on examination, he felt the predominant distortion was a triggerband.

Folding distortions (FDs) of the shoulder can be treated with a variety of maneuvers with or without a thrust at the end, depending on a practitioner's scope of practice. The folding fascia is mobilized so that the altered pleats of folding fascia are straightened out. The proper direction of treatment depends on the mechanism of injury, and should recreate the motion that caused injury. Treatment of FDs should not hurt. If the patient reports pain when a maneuver is being performed then the treatment is being

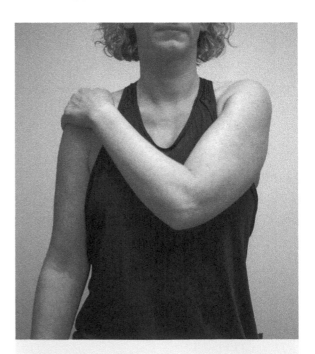

FIGURE 11.26
Patient gesture indicating presence and location of a folding distortion (FD)

performed in the wrong direction and the direction of treatment should be reversed. If this also causes pain, either one of the painful distortions is present in the shoulder (triggerband, HTP, CD, or a combination of these), or the direction of force being attempted is incorrect and a different treatment position should be attempted.

Historically, FD treatments have been the most difficult techniques for practitioners to master. Practice is needed with handholds, different techniques, and subtle variations of force to recreate vectors necessary to achieve a successful treatment. The correct vector of force creates no pain for the patient and mobilizes the folding fascial matrix.

Due to the complex nature of the shoulder joint, it is often difficult to be certain which portion of the shoulder's fascial matrix is refolding, and which portion is unfolding when working through the techniques. This is related to the fact that the joint and matrix are three-dimensional, and a force applied to the joint sometimes has a broader impact than expected or desired. The folding techniques described in this section are those routinely taught as part of the Module 1 course. At times, other folding techniques are developed at the bedside to address the patient's unique mechanism of injury. It is through a thorough understanding and mastery of the concepts of the FDM that these "one-off" techniques may become a reality, to the benefit of the patient.

Shoulder refolding distortions (rFDs)

Shoulder refolding distortions (rFDs) may occur when compressive force is applied to the fascial matrix. Refolding of the joint occurs when there is overcompression of the matrix in the presence of torque, preventing the compressed tissue from returning to the neutral position (Fig. 11.27). A patient may describe an rFD by holding their shoulder or drawing a line across the joint. The observant practitioner may notice that patients with rFDs frequently draw this line with their middle finger (Fig. 11.28).

Frog-leg technique

The frog-leg technique can be diagnostic as well as therapeutic and, when applied to the shoulder, is a classic example of one part of the joint unfolding while another portion is refolding. It is critical

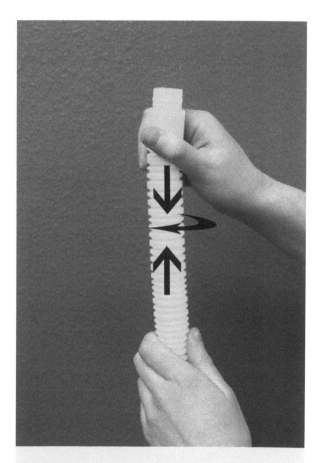

FIGURE 11.27
Shoulder refolding distortion (rFD)

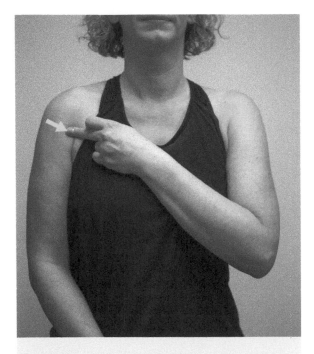

FIGURE 11.28

Patient gesture indicating presence and location of a refolding distortion (rFD)

to remember when treating an FD there should be no pain. If pain is present, force should be applied in the opposite direction, and if there is still pain, then the provider must treat the underlying (painful) distortions before re-attempting the maneuver. The frog-leg (and other folding techniques) may be used to identify underlying painful distortions to address prior to treating the FD.

With this technique, the practitioner stabilizes the elbow with one hand while their other hand grasps the patient's flexed wrist with two fingers above the crease and two fingers below (Fig. 11.29). The elbow is fully flexed, the arm is internally rotated and the wrist is flexed to prevent it from striking the trunk of the patient. When a rotational barrier is reached, a thrust can be performed. The hand placement is then switched (Fig. 11.30). The wrist hand grasps the elbow, and the elbow hand grasps the wrist. The wrist is extended, the elbow continues to be fully flexed, and the arm is externally rotated. Again, when the barrier reached, if the patient has no pain, a small thrust can be applied. The angle of the upper arm

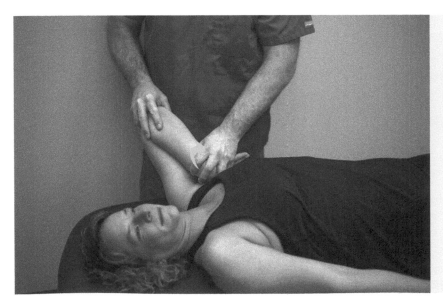

FIGURE 11.29

Frog-leg technique (internal rotation)

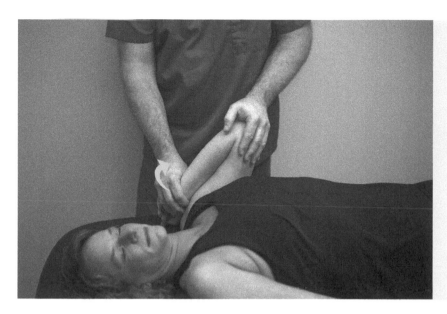

FIGURE 11.30
Frog-leg technique
(external rotation)

during the frog-leg technique is dependent on the patient's input. The practitioner applies the force in the manner that recreates the mechanism of injury, if known, or causes the least discomfort.

If this technique is used to diagnose underlying painful distortions, it can be repeated to determine if the ROM has increased and pain is decreased or resolved.

Shoulder unfolding distortions (uFDs)

Push-out technique

This technique is used to force the upper humerus away from the shoulder. The elbow is stabilized by the practitioner's hand, while the other hand gently grasps the patient's wrist. Force is applied until a barrier is reached (this barrier should not be painful), then a slight thrust or rhythmic thrusting is applied to unfold the tissue. Due to the mechanical structure of the arm, there is a rotational component applied to the humerus when the thrust occurs (Figs. 11.31

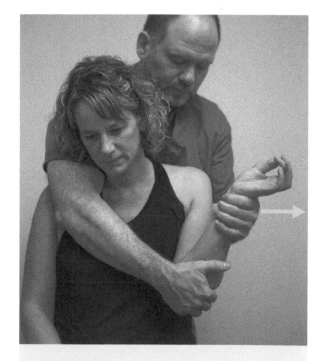

FIGURE 11.31
Push-out technique

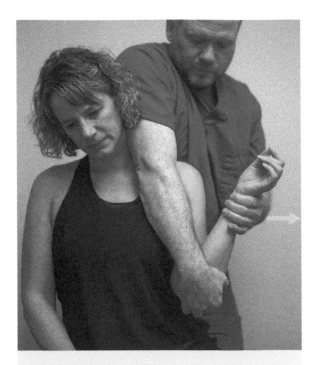

FIGURE 11.32
Push-out technique with alternate hand placement

and 11.32). There are two variations of this technique that can be used depending on practitioner–patient size match-up.

Supine unfolding technique

The supine shoulder unfolding technique can be used to locate the correct vector of force when the mechanism of injury is known. This technique is performed by placing traction on the shoulder in the vector that is least painful, then performing a traction thrust. Some injuries require treatment in multiple vectors to successfully address the injured shoulder. The practitioner may instruct the patient to stabilize themselves by holding onto the table with their other hand, but it is crucial to advise them not to grip too strongly, as this will engage the musculature of the back and shoulder and prevent the

appropriate gapping of the shoulder's fascial matrix (Fig. 11.33). If unfolding treatment along any of the vectors causes pain, it is appropriate to immediately turn the force 180 degrees and direct the force back into the joint to refold the tissue.

Upper arm lever technique (Water Pump)

This variation of the push-out technique was developed to eliminate as much of the humeral rotation as possible. With the lever technique, the practitioner's cephalad forearm is placed between the patient's upper arm and ribs. The practitioner places their caudad forearm on the patient's humerus, elbow to elbow, with fingers positioned at the glenohumeral joint. The practitioner then pushes the patient's elbow in towards their ribs. With the cephalad forearm serving as a fulcrum, the force on the elbow gaps the glenohumoral joint. With proper hand placement, the gapping of the glenohumeral joint can be palpated as the force is applied.

Two different hand positions have been successfully used to perform this maneuver. When levering the patient's humerus over the provider's forearm, the most muscular portion of the provider's forearm must be in contact with the inner portion of the patient's upper arm. The neurovascular bundle on the inside of the upper arm may be compressed by the bone of the practitioner's forearm if an incorrect position is utilized, potentially causing unnecessary discomfort (Figs. 11.34 and 11.35).

Column technique

With all unfolding techniques, adaptations and utilization of one's surroundings may be used to achieve proper force and direction. For example, Dr Typaldos used a column in his office to stabilize a patient's pectoral region while applying a significant amount of traction. Use of a structural column for this purpose will require the application of padding

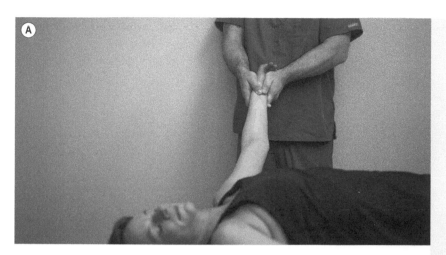

FIGURE 11.33 A–C
Supine shoulder unfolding

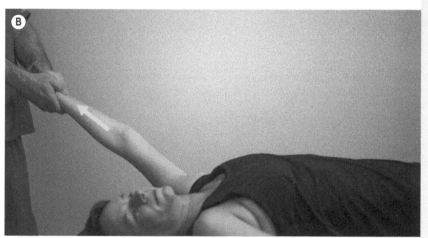

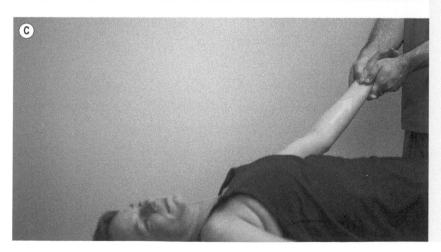

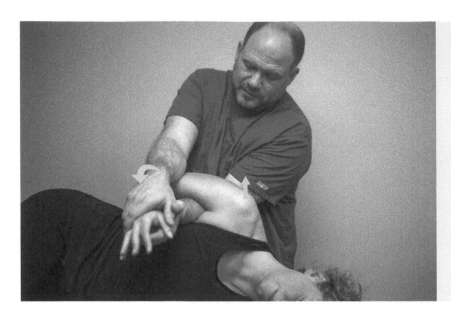

FIGURE 11.34
Upper arm lever technique
(Water Pump)

FIGURE 11.35
Upper arm lever technique
(Water Pump), alternate hand
placement

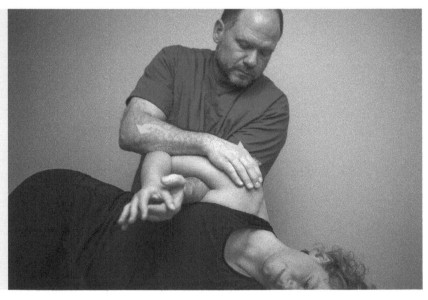

for patient comfort. It is also important to apply steady traction before applying a thrust (Fig. 11.36), Allowing the patient to move away from the column before thrusting would cause their face to be rapidly pulled into the column. Many different vectors can be employed with this technique. Treatment tables that can be raised high off the ground have been utilized for a similar treatment in settings where a column is not readily available. When using the treatment table, it may be helpful to have the patient lie at a diagonal on the table, so when force is applied downward, they do not roll off (Fig. 11.37).

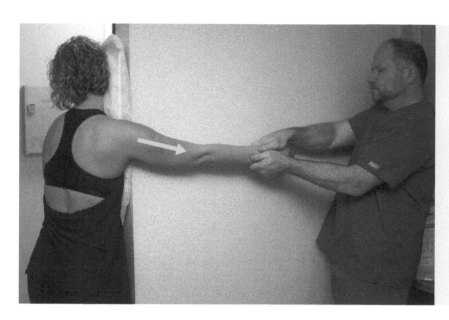

FIGURE 11.36
Column technique

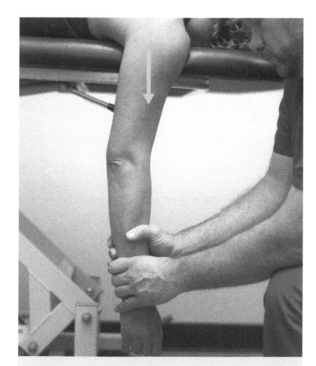

FIGURE 11.37
Column technique on table

Intermuscular septal techniques of the upper arm

It is theorized that all muscles have folding fascia separating them from other muscles. Several prominent septal divisions are regularly treated in the FDM, one being the separation between the biceps and triceps. This intermuscular septum can be both refolded and unfolded. FDs of this area are described with multiple fingers pressing deep into the septum, along the length of the septum (Fig. 11.38). Patients may describe a deep ache that does not have a distinct area of pain, and may also hold their upper arm. Remember, folding treatments do not hurt. Treatment consists of the application of force in the direction of the least amount of pain.

Pump gun technique

This technique involves gripping the bicep in one hand and the triceps in the other (Fig. 11.39A). The two muscles are then moved in opposite directions along the humerus; each muscle moved by the practitioner along the bone until reaching an endpoint. Tension is applied, and if no pain is felt by the

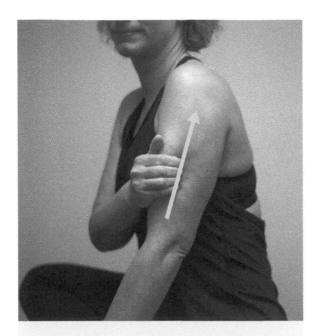

FIGURE 11.38
Fingers pressing deep along the length of the intermuscular septum indicating the presence of a septal folding distortion (FD)

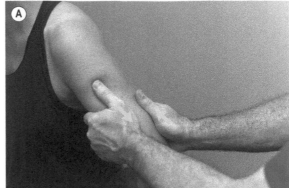

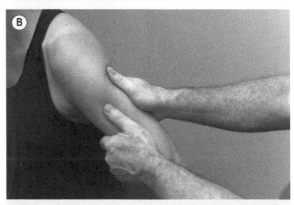

FIGURE 11.39A, B
Pump gun technique

patient, then a thrust can be applied to accentuate the movement. If the patient reports discomfort, then the direction of the force is reversed and the opposing endpoint is reached (Fig. 11.39B). A thrust in this direction is appropriate if no pain is felt.

Chicken wing technique

This technique is performed by grasping the bicep in one hand while supporting the triceps on the thigh of the practitioner. Force is applied to the bicep at a 45-degree angle in a manner that looks like one is trying to shear the biceps muscle from the humerus (Fig. 11.40A). Force is applied in one direction at 45 degrees to the humerus, and if no pain is present, a thrust is performed. If pain is present, then the thrust is performed at 45 degrees in the other direction to the humerus (Fig. 11.40B). If both of these

forces cause pain, the biceps should be grasped from the opposite side and thrust in either direction, again at an angle 45 degrees to the humerus (Figs. 11.40C and D). The correct direction of treatment is in the direction of the least pain when addressing the intermuscular septum of the upper arm.

Anchorage Twist

This maneuver again focuses on the septum located between the biceps and triceps. For this technique, one hand grasps the biceps, and one hand grasps the triceps. It is important that the hand be used as a clamp to stabilize the muscle (Fig. 11.41) but the

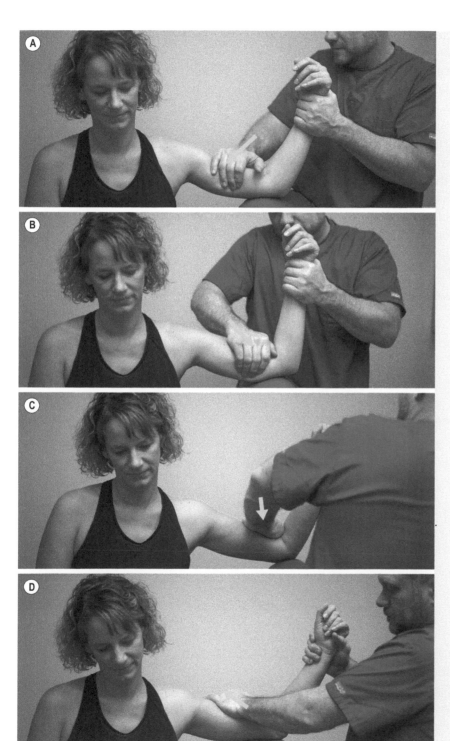

FIGURE 11.40A–D
Chicken wing technique

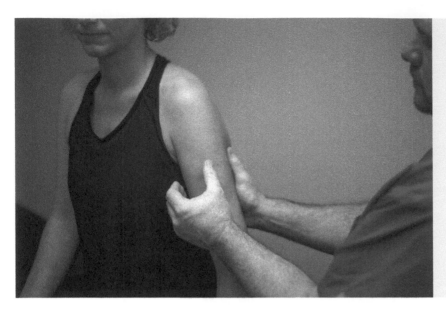

FIGURE 11.41
Anchorage Twist: correct hand placement. Note the fingers are flat against the skin.

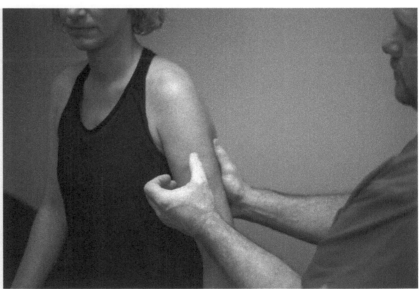

FIGURE 11.42
Anchorage Twist: incorrect hand placement

fingers should not dig into the muscle like claws (Fig. 11.42). With the biceps and triceps stabilized, the patient is then asked to move the hand behind their back as though they are tucking in a shirt or reaching for a bra strap. There is no traction applied to either muscle: the practitioner merely stabilizes the muscles. The force of the patient moving their arm in this way provides the force across the septum (Figs. 11.43 and 11.44).

Jar technique

The jar technique is usually applied in conjunction with the Anchorage Twist. With the arm behind the back, the biceps and triceps are rotated so that the

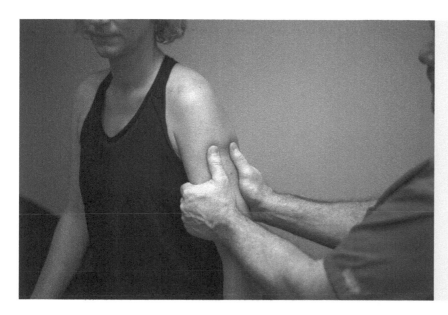

FIGURE 11.43
Anchorage Twist: practitioner stablizes biceps and triceps

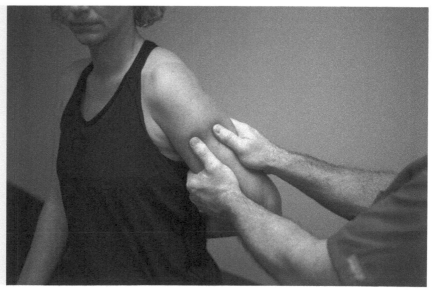

FIGURE 11.44
Anchorage Twist: with upper arm stabilized, patient moves hand behind back

hand presses against the back (Fig. 11.45). A barrier is reached, and if not painful, a thrust applied. The patient's palm is then placed on their abdomen, and rotational force applied so that the hand moves toward their stomach (Fig. 11.46). Again, if the rotation does not cause pain, then a thrust is applied.

Cylinder distortions (CyDs) of the shoulder

Cylinder distortions (CyDs) of the shoulder region are described by the patient squeezing, sweeping, or wiping the area of complaint. Often patients describe pain of inexplicable intensity or that the pain appears

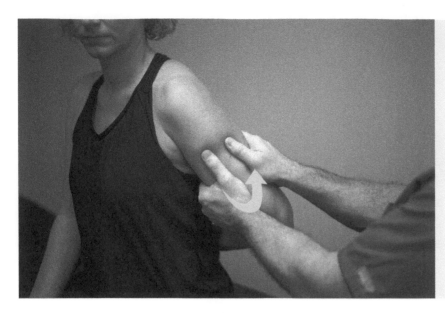

FIGURE 11.45
Jar technique: rotational
thrust applied

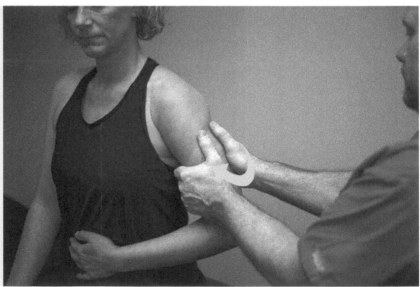

FIGURE 11.46
Jar technique: rotational
thrust applied in opposite
direction

to jump from one location to another. The symptoms of CyD are bizarre and may confuse the practitioner since the pain does not appear to follow traditional anatomical distributions or referral patterns. The cause of CyDs is thought to be a tangle in the most superficial fascial coils of the fascial matrix. When treating a CyD, the skin overlying the distortion is either stabilized or pulled away from the underlying fascia in an attempt to untangle the fascial coils.

Many modalities can be used to treat CyDs. These can be divided into manipulative and non-manipulative techniques. Manipulative techniques use the practitioner's hands to mobilize the skin in

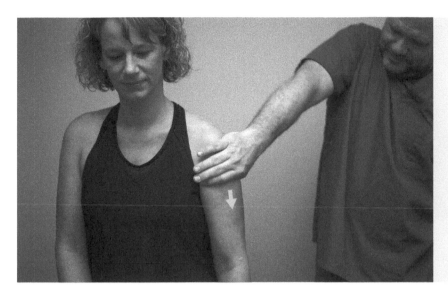

FIGURE 11.47
Squeegee technique

such a manner that separates the tangled coils of fascia, while non-manipulative techniques employ various devices to untangle the coils.

Squeegee technique

When performing the squeegee technique on the shoulder area, the edge of the thumb and index finger are rubbed along the skin as if trying to remove water from the surface of the skin. The pressure applied forces the tangled coils to untangle (Fig. 11.47).

Double-thumb technique

When using the double-thumb technique, the thumbs are pressed into the tissue and then separated. The focus of the force is not a sliding motion across the skin, but rather the separation of the superficial fibers below the skin. When traction is applied with double-thumb technique, constant pressure on the fascial coils results in a palpable stretch of the fascia. The double-thumb technique may also be first applied in one direction and then in the other. This technique can be used to cover any size cylinder distortion, but as it is labor-intensive it is generally used on smaller cylinder distortions (Fig. 11.48).

Cupping with movement

This technique is performed by placing a cup over the area identified as a CyD and applying a small-to-moderate amount of suction. The patient then moves the shoulder through a ROM. One or more cups may be used and the size of the cup can be determined by the size of the CyD(s) described. The arm and shoulder should be moved in all directions with the cup in place (Fig. 11.49).

Cupping with sliding

In this technique, a cup is placed on the skin after a slight amount of lubricating lotion is applied and then slid across the skin. As the cup moves across the skin, the skin is separated from the superficial fascial coils, allowing them to uncoil.

Vacuum extractor technique

The vacuum extractor is a device that is used in obstetrics to secure a baby's head and assist the mother in delivering the child through the birth canal. This same tool can be used to distract the skin while the patient moves, or it can be slid along the

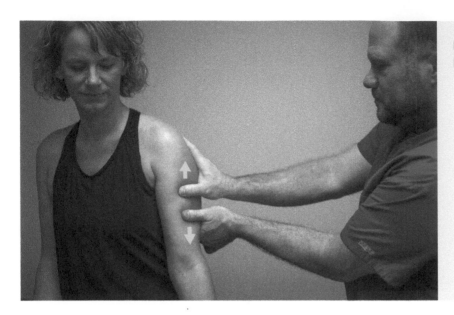

FIGURE 11.48
Double-thumb technique

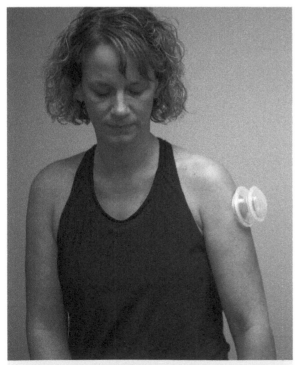

FIGURE 11.49
Cupping with movement

skin; convenient when the CyD is present in larger areas of skin (Fig. 11.50).

Plunger technique

The plunger can be considered to be a very large cup for purposes of treatment of CyDs. Using a plunger allows for treatment of larger areas in a single application. As with smaller cups, the plunger can be used to pull the skin away from the underlying fascial coils.

Using the plunger technique for FDs of the scapula

The fascia between the scapula and the posterior ribs acts as folding fascia. When this fascia is overcompressed, and a torque force occurs, a refolding of the scapula has occurred. This is treated with rhythmic compression of the scapula against the posterior ribs in many different directions. Since this a folding injury, the correct direction of treatment is in the direction that does not cause pain (Fig. 11.51).

Any tissue that can refold, by definition, can unfold. Any force that causes the scapula to pull away from the posterior ribs with the addition of

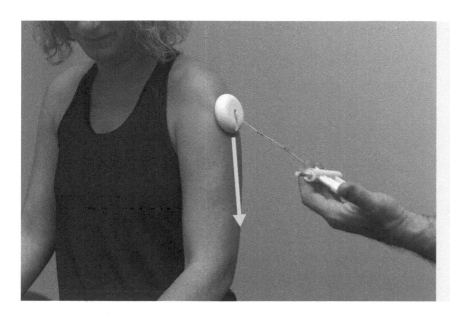

FIGURE 11.50
Vacuum extractor technique employed for cupping with sliding

FIGURE 11.51
Treatment of scapular refolding distortions (rFDs)

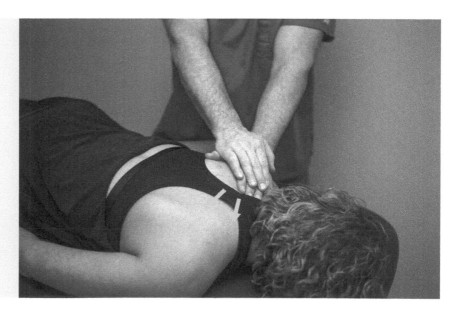

torque, preventing the scapula from moving back to the neutral position, is a uFD. This distortion is treated by pulling the scapula away from the posterior ribs. This can be accomplished using the plunger to distract and mobilize the scapula in many different directions (Fig. 11.52).

Shoulder tectonic fixations (TFs)

Any fascial surface may become tectonic. In the shoulder, the glenohumeral joint and the scapula are two common tectonic fixations (TFs). When a TF occurs, fascial surfaces become stuck together and

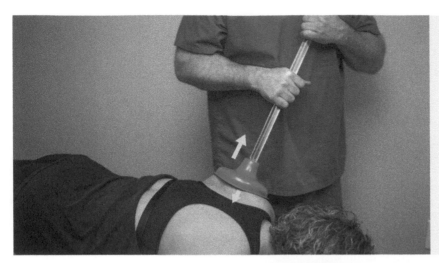

FIGURE 11.52
Plunger technique for treatment of scapular unfolding distortions (uFDs)

FIGURE 11.53A, B
Tectonic pump of the shoulder

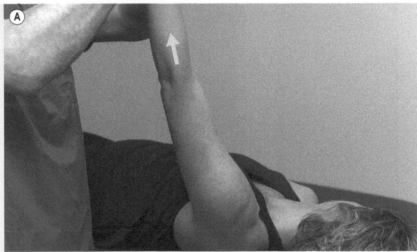

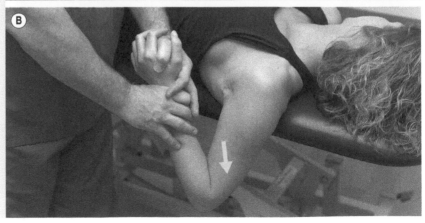

are unable to slide against each other, restricting the movement of the fascial matrix. TFs are not painful: since the fascial layers are not moving against one another, there is no perception of pain. Instead, they represent a global loss of ROM.

When the fascial layers of the glenohumeral joint become stuck together, the practitioner must increase the fluid between the layers. First, the fluid in the joint can be made less viscous by applying heat before the treatment. This is the only distortion where heat is recommended as part of the treatment. Next, the shoulder is put through a slow tectonic pump, achieved by moving the shoulder to the extent of flexion and extension. When a barrier is reached, the pressure is held, encouraging the matrix to stretch while fluid seeps between the layers. Stretching and holding the shoulder in multiple planes encourages the fluid to be moved between different fascial layers. As the patient identifies painful distortions, they should be treated and eliminated. A continued slow tectonic technique is performed after treating a painful distortion, maximizing the ROM and fluid movement (Fig. 11.53). This tectonic pump

concept can be applied to any tissue that is thought to be experiencing a TF.

Frog-leg technique

Frog-leg technique can be used to apply rotational force into a TF in the shoulder. This technique is often combined with flexion and extension of the shoulder in a slow rhythmic pressure on the fascial matrix.

Brute force technique

Brute force technique can be applied to separate the fascial layers of the glenohumeral joint. In this technique, the practitioner is positioned behind the patient, and the heels of the practitioner's hands are placed on the glenohumeral junction. Direct downward traction followed by a thrust is used to separate the fascial layers (Fig. 11.54).

TF of the scapula

The scapula may become tectonically fixed to the thoracic region when the fascia between the scapula and posterior ribs becomes immobile and stuck.

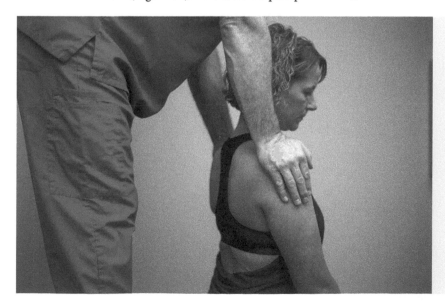

FIGURE 11.54
Brute force treatment directed at glenohumeral joint

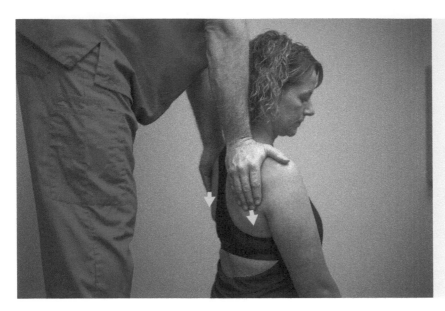

FIGURE 11.55
Brute force treatment
directed at scapula

This adhesion, or fixed fascia, may be treated using the plunger to rhythmically pump fluid between the fascial layers. The plunger is applied to the scapula, and the scapula is lifted from the rib cage in a slow pumping motion. Additionally, the scapula can be moved from side to side with the hands to put tension on the fixed fascial layers. The brute force technique can be adapted so that the provider's force is shearing the scapula away from the posterior ribs (Fig. 11.55).

The distortions found in the hand are the same as those found elsewhere in the body. It is not uncommon for distortions in the hand to extend into the arm, or for distortions in the arm to extend into the hand.

Digital triggerbands

Finger triggerbands are a frequent occurrence, but they can and do occur elsewhere in the hands. As with all triggerbands, they are wherever the patient identifies them. Care should be taken when observing patients with complaints of hand pain, since the triggerband can be quite small and easy to misdiagnose as a different distortion such as a continuum distortion (CD) (Fig. 12.1).

Herniated triggerpoints (HTPs) of the hand

The size of herniated trigger points (HTPs) in the hand may be much smaller than in other regions. The patient gesture and verbal description used by

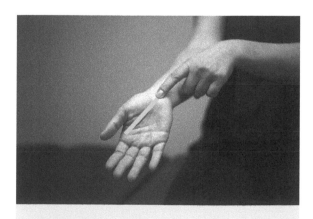

FIGURE 12.1
Palmar triggerband (TB)

the practitioner to diagnose the distortion remains the same, however, as does the treatment. As smaller distortions often require less force to treat, it is not uncommon for hand HTPs to respond to a smaller amount of pressure. With a smaller target, the focus of force becomes critical, as does overall technique.

Continuum distortions (CDs) of the hand

These distortions are often very small, but no less problematic for the patient. Palpatory skill is beneficial when identifying and treating these, sometimes tiny, distortions. As usual with CDs, this is an all-or-nothing treatment, and focused force and technique are critical. Palpation of the CD release helps minimize the pain that is experienced by the patient and reduces the overall treatment time required to establish improvement in range of movement (ROM) and function.

Folding distortions (FDs) of the hand

As with other distortions in the hand, folding gestures may be much more subtle and easily confused. When a patient holds their hand to explain the location of the pain, many small joints could be included in that simple gesture (Fig. 12.2).

Cylinder distortions (CyDs) of the hand

Sweeping of the hand or squeezing of the fingers is a good indication of a cylinder distortion (CyD). Bizarre, unusual symptoms or any unusual sensation in the hand are also a good indication. Manipulative techniques – like the squeegee and double-thumb – lend themselves nicely to the small area and contours

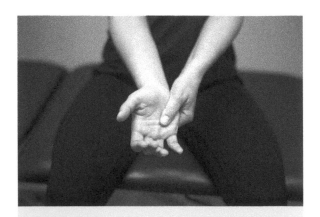

FIGURE 12.2
Gesture indicating the presence of a folding distortion (FD) in the hand

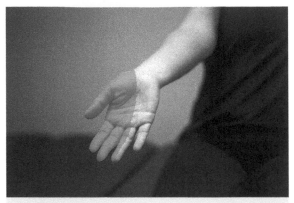

FIGURE 12.3
Common distribution of carpal tunnel syndrome (CTS) symptoms

of the hand, although small cups may also be used on dorsal or palmar aspects.

Tectonic fixations (TFs) of the hand

Any joint or fascial surface may develop a tectonic fixation (TF). Prolonged immobilization in a cast or splint can lead to tectonically-fixed joints in the hand resulting in the joints feeling stiff and like they need to "pop". There is loss of range of motion (ROM) and fixed areas will not be tender upon palpation. This is the only distortion that is heated before treatment. Once heated, a pump technique can be utilized to increase fluid movement between the layers of tectonically-fixed fascia.

Carpal tunnel syndrome

This condition can be treated effectively using the FDM as a guide. It is important to differentiate between carpal tunnel syndrome (CTS) and carpal tunnel-like syndrome (CTLS). The difference between these syndromes is a positive electromyography (EMG), indicating compression of the median nerve in CTS (Fig. 12.3). In cases of CTS, it is critical to discuss the importance of close monitoring of

hand strength with the patient. Monitoring for and identifying any weakness or atrophy of the hand muscles would prompt a recommendation for surgical intervention and if there is evidence of thenar eminence atrophy, surgical evaluation is recommended. A positive EMG does not preclude treatment using the FDM, but it should be used in conjunction with close monitoring due to the risk of permanent injury. When a patient understands the symptoms to watch for and the possible ramifications of ignoring them, the treatment of CTS and CTLS is essentially the same, and it is not uncommon for FDM treatment to provide relief for patients with CTS.

A diagnosis of CTS is predicated on compression of the median nerve with associated numbness or neurologic change in the distribution of the median nerve. This is generally described as the thumb, index finger, middle finger, and the radial half of the ring finger. The general mechanism is thought to be that of congestion of the carpal tunnel and surgical correction of CTS involves cutting the flexor retinaculum to release pressure and restriction of the median nerve. It is important to watch the patient's description of their pain and treat what they demonstrate as the source of the problem when working in the FDM. Often, CyDs are described, and these should be treated.

Treatment of many triggerbands, both parallel to and perpendicular to the flexor retinaculum should be performed (Figs. 12.4). Treating the dorsal aspect of the tunnel using triggerband technique can also free up the flexor retinaculum (Fig. 12.5). Mobilization of the wrist and carpals can address unfolding (uFDs) and refolding distortions (rFDs) of the wrist and

hand. Unfolding of the carpal tunnel once the flexor retinaculum has been released can provide relief. Unfolding of the interosseous membrane of the wrist is performed by the practitioner placing their thumbs on the radial and ulnar styloid and generating a force that unfolds the membrane between the two bones, opening the tunnel (Figs. 12.6 and 12.7). This folding treatment can be performed with the practitioner's thumbs crossed, or with the thumbs parallel in the canal, providing lateral pressure.

While these are standard techniques employed in patients experiencing both CTS and CTLS, it is imperative to watch the patient and allow them to guide the treatment.

Triggerband thumb

Dr Typaldos identified triggerband thumb as a condition that develops in a practitioner treating triggerbands. It is thought to be associated with the development of triggerbands and rFDs in the thumb, and is caused by the pressure needed to treat triggerbands. Self-treatment of these distortions can decrease the pain in the practitioner's thumb and

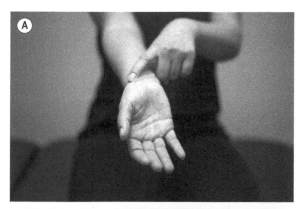

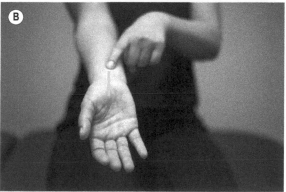

FIGURE 12.4A, B
Triggerbands associated with carpal tunnel syndrome (CTS)

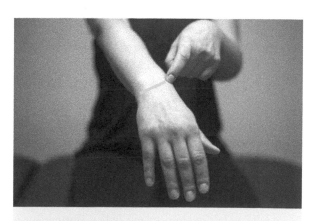

FIGURE 12.5
Triggerband on dorsal aspect of wrist

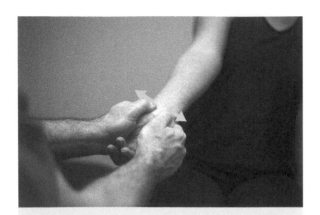

FIGURE 12.6
Unfolding the interosseous membrane of the wrist

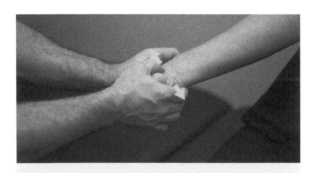

FIGURE 12.7
Unfolding the interosseous membrane of the wrist, alternate thumb placement

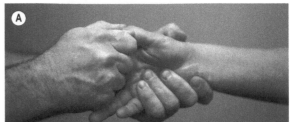

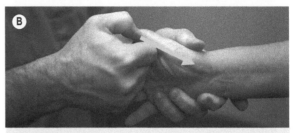

FIGURE 12.8 A, B
Treating triggerband thumb

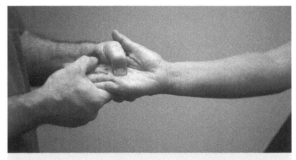

FIGURE 12.9
Correcting distortions along the trigger finger's flexor tendon

restore the power the practitioner can apply when treating patients (Fig. 12.8).

Trigger finger

In the medical realm, trigger finger is thought to be due to a dysfunction of the pulley system in the finger. In the FDM, careful attention to the gestures described by a patient can guide the treatment. It is not uncommon to see triggerbands and CDs associated with the tendon and pulley involved. Focused, attentive treatment can improve the function of the tendon/pulley system (Fig. 12.9).

Jammed finger

The jammed finger is an analogy that is commonly used to help students of the FDM understand FDs.

A common scenario involves a finger joint getting jammed or compressed during sporting activity; for example, a ball impacts a player's fingertip on an axial vector, rapidly compressing the joints in the finger, causing a refolding injury. The typical reaction to this type of injury is for practitioners to pull on the finger, demonstrating a failure to understand FDs. Instead, the injury needs to be recreated to fix the refolded fascia, in other words, the finger needs to be compressed and, at the same time, a rotational force added to find the vector where the refolding occurred. The correct vector is found by twisting the finger in the least painful direction. Remember that FDs should not hurt to treat.

Dupuytren's contracture

By listening to the description of the patient's complaints and watching their gestures, Dupuytren's contracture can be addressed in the FDM. Common distortions found in Dupuytren's contracture include TFs, triggerbands, CDs, and HTPs (Fig. 12.10). Treatment appears to slow the development of further scarring, but the frequency and number of treatments required for each patient to have symptom relief is unknown at this time. Patients can be taught to treat the distortions they identify in their hands, but self-treatment is often limited due to how painful treatment is.

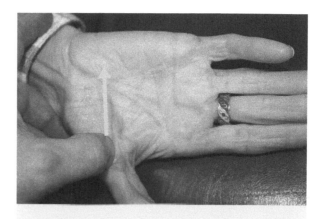

FIGURE 12.10
Treatment of palmar contracture with triggerband technique

In the elbow region of the upper extremity, as in all other regions of the body, observation of the patient's pain gesture will guide the practitioner to the location of triggerbands, continuum distortions (CDs), and herniated trigger points (HTPs).

Elbow folding distortions (FDs)

Folding distortions (FDs) of the elbow are treated as in any other region. Unfold the unfolding distortions (uFDs) and refold the refolding distortions (rFDs),

and always remember the treatment of FDs should not hurt. Patient feedback, specifically whether or not they feel pain, will guide the treatment.

The frog-leg test can be diagnostic as well as therapeutic for FDs in the elbow (Fig. 13.1). Mobilization of the elbow to induce unfolding and refolding is the essence of this treatment. The technique can also be used for tectonic fixations (TFs) as it mobilizes fascial layers and pumps fluid into the elbow joint.

When a patient is holding the radial head, this can represent either a uFD or an rFD of the radial head (Fig. 13.2).

Radial head unfolding distortions (uFDs)

In this treatment, the patient is placed supine with their arm resting on the table. The palm of one of the practitioner's hands cups the AC joint, pressing the shoulder towards the table. Care should be used as this area of the anterior shoulder can be painful if

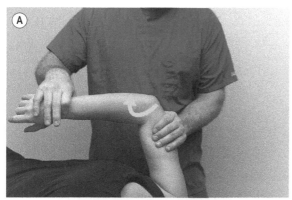

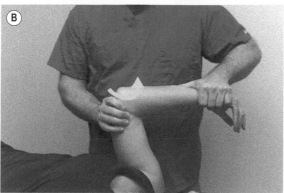

Figure 13.1 A, B
Application of the frog-leg technique to the elbow

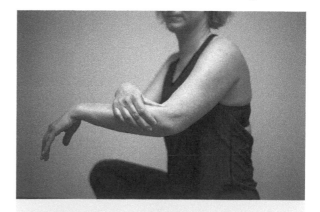

FIGURE 13.2
Patient gesture indicating presence and location of folding distortion (FD) in the elbow region

palpated too aggressively. The pressure applied to the shoulder raises the patient's forearm off the table, with the elbow acting as a fulcrum, and the practitioner's other hand grasps the patient's wrist. Adjustment of the angle of the forearm engages different planes of tissue. At the point of greatest comfort, the wrist is tractioned and a thrust is applied towards the table, unfolding the radial head (Fig. 13.3).

Radial head refolding distortions (rFDs)

If the patient draws a line across the radial head or describes pain with techniques used to unfold the radial head, then refolding of the radial head can be performed. This technique should not cause pain. Various force vectors may need to be applied to get the proper refolding to occur (Fig. 13.4).

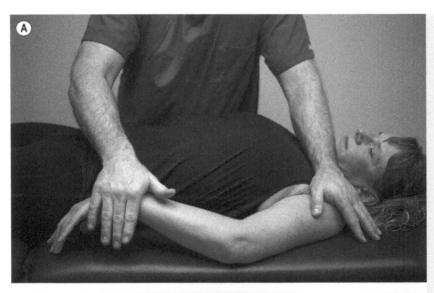

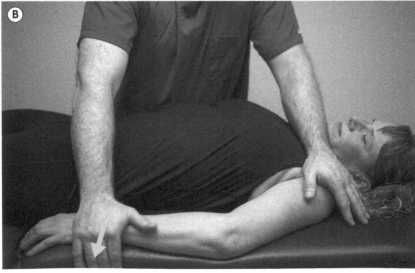

FIGURE 13.3A, B
Unfolding treatment of radial head

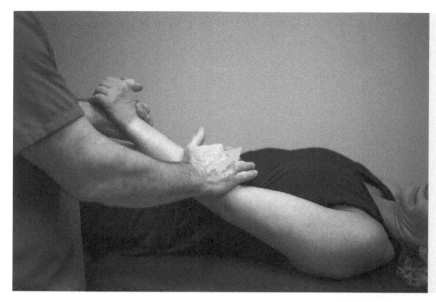

FIGURE 13.4
Refolding treatment of radial head

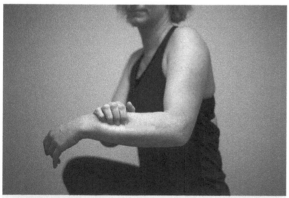

FIGURE 13.5
Patient gesture indicating presence and location of folding distortion (FD) of the interosseous membrane

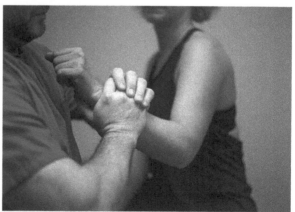

FIGURE 13.6
Refolding treatment of interosseous membrane

Interosseous membrane folding distortions (FDs)

The interosseous membrane of the forearm is the membrane located between the radius and the ulna. The patient will describe a deep ache between the bones and demonstrates this ache by pressing multiple fingers into area between the radius and ulna (Fig. 13.5). The membrane between these bones is thought to have fibers that run 45 degrees to the bone. If a patient presents with pain deep in the forearm and the diagnosis of an interosseous membrane folding is suspected, the radius and ulna can be compressed together to refold this membrane (Fig. 13.6). If this is painful, the membrane may need to be unfolded. When unfolding the membrane, many different vectors may need to be applied to get the proper correction of the folded fascia, directed by treating in the direction that does not hurt. The aim of the practitioner is to separate the radius and ulna with a force that is 45 degrees to the bone. The heel of the hand is placed on one of the bones, and pressure applied to separate it from the other bone. Constant shifting of force vectors helps fine-tune the treatments (Fig. 13.7).

Tiger claw technique

The tiger claw technique can be used to mobilize tissue deep in the interosseous membrane of the forearm. This can be used to address both FDs and TFs.

This technique is performed by grasping the skin on the dorsal aspect of the forearm, before putting the through a range of motion (ROM). Often a deep ache is noted as the interosseous tissue is moved, but treatment should not be painful (Fig. 13.8).

Cylinder distortions (CyDs)

Both manual and mechanical techniques can be used to correct cylinder distortions (CyDs) of the upper extremity. Care should be used, as this area is prone to the formation of CyDs, and overtreatment may cause more CyDs. The ease of CyD formation in this area can be seen by the frequency of unusual pains in the

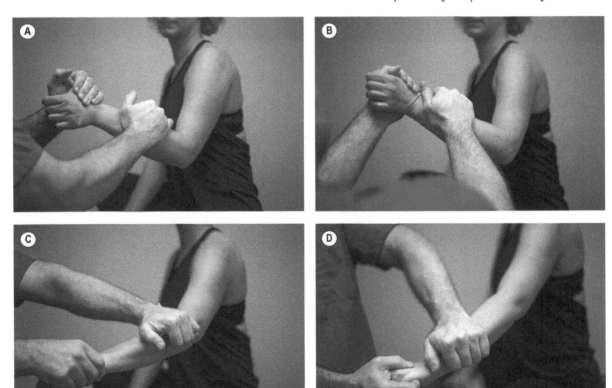

FIGURE 13.7A–D
Unfolding treatment of interosseous membrane

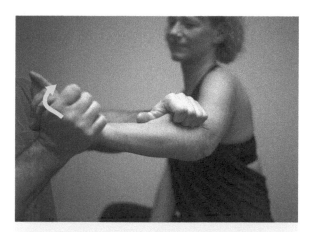

FIGURE 13.8

Tiger claw technique with wrist movement

arm following medication injection. It is thought that coiled or circular fascia twist or kink when punctured with a needle, causing a CyD. In patients with extreme symptoms following an injection in this region, the practitioner can often relieve pain by performing CyD correction techniques such as the double-thumb.

Epicondylitis

This commonly diagnosed condition can be very effectively treated in the FDM. Close observation of the patient's gesture will lead the practitioner to the proper distortion diagnosis. Triggerbands and CDs are the most commonly associated distortions associated with epicondylitis, although all six distortions may contribute to the condition.

When dealing with the wrist and conditions found here, the patient guides the practitioner as usual. All distortions can be found in the wrist. Proper diagnosis and treatment is achieved through careful observation and attention to the patient's description of their pain.

De Quervain's tenosynovitis-like pain

Pain in the dorsal or radial distribution of the thumb is routinely diagnosed as De Quervain's tenosynovitis. Classic diagnostic criteria are a tight, pulling, burning sensation from the thumb up the radial aspect of the wrist (Fig. 14.1). Practitioners of the Fascial Distortion Model (FDM) will recognize this distribution as a triggerband. Whichever distortion is identified by the patient,

treatment can provide significant relief for this condition.

Wrist folding distortions (FDs)

Wrist pain that presents with the patient holding the joint and experiencing pain deep in the joint is consistent with a folding distortion (FD) of the wrist (Fig. 14.2). The wrist can unfold or refold in a multitude of directions. As folding treatments do not hurt, the wrist can be mobilized with repeated unfolding and refolding to alter the three-dimensional fascial tissue and return it to normal function (Fig. 14.3).

Refolding of the wrist can be achieved by using the patient's hand to refold the wrist joint. Again, this should not be painful (Fig. 14.4).

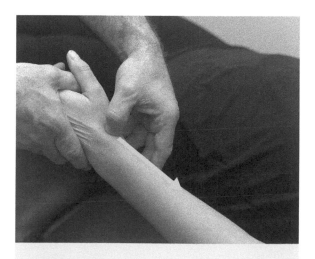

FIGURE 14.1
Triggerband technique applied to the wrist

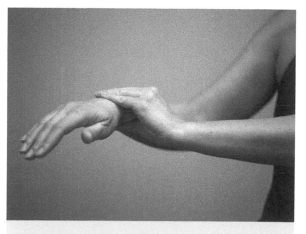

FIGURE 14.2
Patient gesture indicating presence and location of a folding distortion (FD)

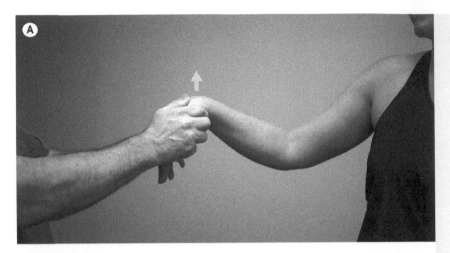

FIGURE 14.3A–C
Wrist mobilization for folding distortion (FD) treatment

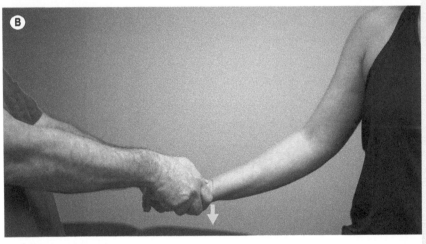

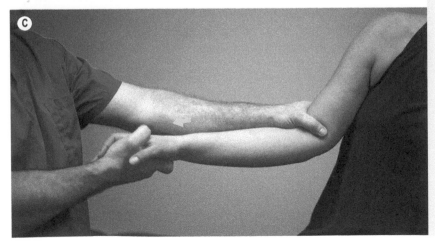

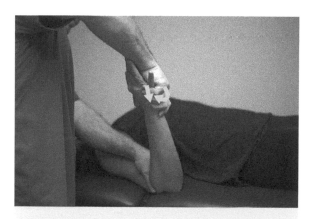

FIGURE 14.4
Compression with mobilization for refolding distortion (rFD) in wrist

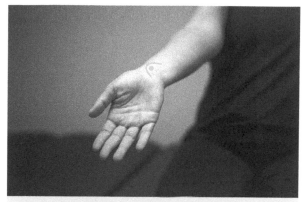

FIGURE 14.5
Continuum distortions (CDs) and triggerbands can be found around ganglion cysts

Ganglion cysts

Ganglion cysts are incredibly common, and they can also be treated in the FDM. Ganglion cysts are thought to arise from the accumulation of fluid in dense connective tissue, along with formation of a valve-like structure. Some form of stricture affects the patency of the valve, preventing fluid from draining. When treating these cysts, watching the gesture provided by the patient may direct the practitioner to the cause of the outflow obstruction. In the absence of a clear gesture, an altered piece of banded fascia may to be the cause of dysfunction in the cyst's normal draining mechanism. Since this occurs in banded fascia, the two distortions found in banded fascia (CDs located at either end of the altered band of fascia, or triggerbands found within the banded fascia) can be treated. Addressing both these distortions may improve the symptoms of the ganglion cyst (Fig. 14.5)

Ankle

As with any region of the body, the practitioner should create their own standardized assessment of the region. Having a standard evaluation of the ankle that includes dorsiflexion, plantarflexion, heel walking, toe walking, walking on the outside of the foot, squatting on toes, and squatting with heels flat, ensures that the full ankle motion is evaluated. Doing this for each ankle injury as it is encountered enables a practitioner to build a body of knowledge for comparison.

When evaluating an ankle sprain, adherence to the Ottawa Criteria for ankle radiography or Ottawa Ankle Rules (OAR) (Fig. 15.1) helps to decide whether an X-ray of an ankle injury is clinically indicated. Developed by Canadian emergency physician Ian Stiell and his research team in 1992, the Ottawa Ankle Rules have been found to be nearly 100% sensitive for ruling out the presence of ankle and midfoot fractures (Bachman, et al., 2003). The Rules have been repeatedly validated for use in adults, and use in children age 2 to 16 has also been validated (Plint, et al., 1999). While validated, Dr Stiell (2019) advises caution when applying the rules to children.

> **Ottawa Rules**
>
> To assess a patient's ankle with the Ottawa Rules:
>
> 1. Assess whether the patient can bear weight on the injured ankle
>
> 2. If patient can bear weight, palpate
>
>   a. Posterior aspects of medial and lateral malleoli
>
>   b. The base of the 5th metatarsal
>
>   c. The navicular bone
>
> 3. If any of these are painful, an X-ray is indicated
>
> If a practitioner's scope of practice allows treatment of fractures, the X-ray can be obtained following the FDM treatment. If a practitioner's scope prevents them from treating fractures, an X-ray should be obtained before the treatment of the injury.

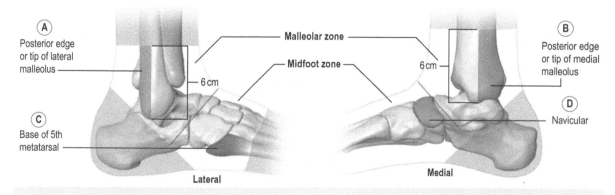

FIGURE 15.1
Ottawa Criteria for ankle radiography
© 1992 et 2013, Institut de recherche de l'Hôpital d'Ottawa, reproduced with kind permission of Dr Ian Stiell

Anterior ankle continuum distortions (AACDs)

Ankle pain and ankle injuries are quite common and are an excellent example of how the Fascial Distortion Model (FDM) can change the paradigm of traditional healthcare. Standard medical care of ankle sprains usually involves splinting, icing, and weeks of rest. With FDM treatment, patients may return to activity the same day as treatment. In the FDM, the goal is to treat the fascial distortion, mobilize the patient, and return them to normal function (or as close to normal as possible).

Dr Typaldos stated that every ankle sprain had an anterior ankle continuum distortion (AACD) present. Locating and treating the AACD is imperative to the complete treatment of the sprained ankle. While AACDs (and the associated gesture) may not be present in every ankle injury, it is crucial to locate this distortion and treat it, restoring dorsiflexion of the ankle. In some cases, restoring dorsiflexion of the ankle is all that is necessary to allow a patient to resume a physiologic walking pattern. Pre- and post-ROM testing is a good way to monitor the effectiveness of the FDM treatment. Restoration of normal gait allows for the correction of the other distortions present in the injured ankle.

The AACD is typically located in the anterior joint line of the ankle, on the distal tibial or talar surface of the mortise joint (Fig. 15.2). The patient will identify the precise location of the CD by identifying the most painful spot palpated. Applying pressure from the bony tip of the practitioner's thumb directly onto the calcific transition zone of the CD resets the transition zone. To the practitioner, the AACD represents a small calcific spot on the periosteum of the bone, thought to be a sharp angulated piece of calcium that needs to be shifted back into the transition zone of the continuum. Correction of the AACD often provides significant improvement in the dorsiflexion and plantar flexion of the ankle (Fig. 15.3).

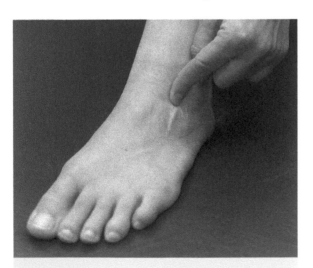

FIGURE 15.2
Gesture indicating presence and location of anterior ankle continuum distortion (AACD)

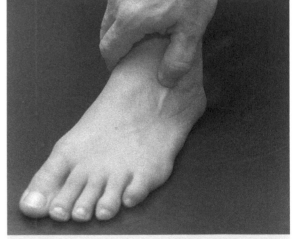

FIGURE 15.3
Treatment of anterior ankle continuum distortion (AACD) with continuum technique

Types of ankle sprains

Once the AACD has been corrected, the type of ankle sprain can be determined. Dr Typaldos identified four types of ankle sprains: the continuum sprain, triggerband sprain, refolding sprain, and the unfolding sprain. These can be identified not only by the mechanism of injury, but the visual appearance of the injured ankle.

Continuum sprained ankle

Lateral ankle sprains, in which sudden inversion of the ankle cause causes immediate pain on the outside of the ankle, are the most common sprain (Doherty, et al., 2013). This mechanism can be thought of as the "stepped-off-the-curb-wrong" ankle sprain. When this sprain occurs, the force of the inversion causes supination of the foot and strain on the lateral aspect of the ankle, and the sudden occurrence of the stress causes CDs. These ankle sprains will have visible swelling over the lateral aspect of the ankle and patients may identify multiple discrete points of pain using a single finger. Appropriate treatment is continuum technique (Fig. 15.4).

Triggerband sprained ankle

Triggerband sprained ankle generally occurs when there is a sudden inversion and torsion of the ankle, for example when a person twists their ankle and falls towards the same side. Dr Typaldos identified this as the "tripped-down-the-stairs" ankle sprain. The torque applied in this mechanism is transmitted up through the ankle into the calf. Often a pulling is felt, and patients may report hearing a "snap". These sprains commonly develop ecchymosis over the ankle and in the foot. Patients will identify their pain with a sweeping of the fingers over the lateral leg, ankle, and foot. Visible swelling is often present over the lateral ankle. This type of sprain is treated with triggerband technique following the correction of the AACD (Fig. 15.5).

Unfolding sprained ankle

Unfolding sprained ankle occurs when a person's foot is held in place and a gapping of the mortise joint occurs in conjunction with a twist or eversion, and

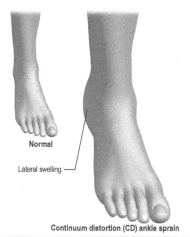

FIGURE 15.4
Continuum distortion (CD) sprained ankle

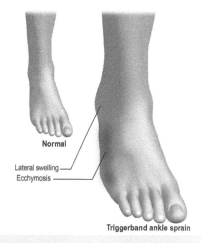

FIGURE 15.5
Triggerband sprained ankle

can be associated with a "shoestring tackle" mechanism. Dr Typaldos identified this as the "stepped-on-the-foot" ankle sprain. Visually, these sprains are often accompanied by an impressive amount of bilateral swelling. The pain identified by the patient is deep in the joint, and the patient is often unable to identify specific spots of pain. They may gesture to the whole ankle, or they may hold the ankle when asked to describe the location of the pain. These sprains will be treated with unfolding technique. It is not uncommon for patients to express that the ankle feels like it needs to "pop" (Fig. 15.6).

Refolding sprained ankle

Refolding sprained ankle is a common presentation to the FDM practitioner. This injury occurs when the foot is forcibly driven into the mortise joint. Dr Typaldos uses the example of misjudging the last step at the end of a flight of stairs, jamming the foot into the ankle, and so refers to these sprains as the "missed-a-step" ankle sprain. The patient will again hold the ankle when asked to demonstrate the

location of their pain, and may use a finger (often the middle finger) to draw a line across the ankle joint. The swelling may be bilateral and will often be less significant than in an unfolding sprained ankle. Treatment of these sprains will require refolding technique. This type of injury is thought to present less often because the patient is repeatedly refolding the ankle with every step they make (Fig. 15.7).

These four types of ankle sprains represent the purest forms of sprain but it is not uncommon for a patient to have a mixture of distortions within an injury, although a single distortion may be the most prominent. A patient will guide the practitioner through treatment by identifying the next distortion that is causing them pain as each distortion is resolved. By listening, watching, and treating what the patient demonstrates, significant improvement in ROM and function can occur. FDM treatment of ankle sprains often eliminates the need for splints, crutches, and rest. In fact, the use of these modalities following FDM treatment may slow the healing process.

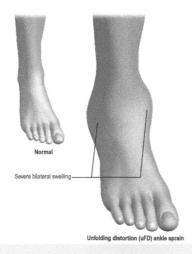

Normal

Severe bilateral swelling

Unfolding distortion (uFD) ankle sprain

FIGURE 15.6
Unfolding distortion (uFD) sprained ankle

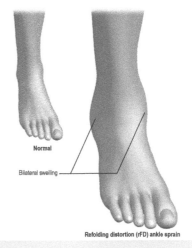

Normal

Bilateral swelling

Refolding distortion (rFD) ankle sprain

FIGURE 15.7
Refolding distortion (rFD) sprained ankle

Ankle triggerbands

The most critical point when addressing trigger-bands in the ankle is to remember that they occur wherever a patient identifies them. A patient will use one or more fingers to draw a line that represents the location of their pain. This sweeping motion is the exact location of the distorted fascial band. They may describe a burning, pulling pain or the sensation of tightness. Triggerbands may be associated with instability of the joint they surround, significant bruising or ecchymosis. Triggerbands are painful along the entire pathway when being treated.

Lateral ankle triggerband

The most common triggerband in ankle sprains is the lateral ankle triggerband. This usually begins near midcalf and then travels to the lateral malleolus, frequently passing below the malleolus, onto the dorsal foot, and out one of the toes. When treating this triggerband, following the pain the patient describes is crucial to successful treatment. During treatment the pain may "headlight" or broadcast down the triggerband, as evidenced by a patient describing pain distal to the location of the practitioner's thumb (Fig. 15.8).

Medial ankle triggerband

See Fig. 15.9.

Anterior ankle triggerband

See Fig. 15.10.

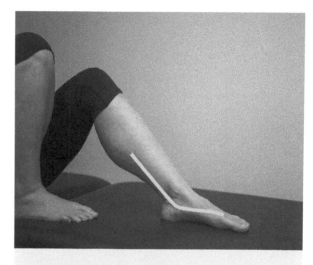

FIGURE 15.9
Medial ankle triggerband

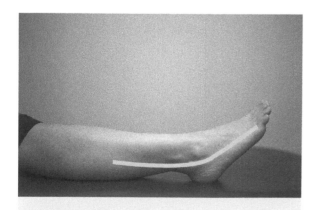

FIGURE 15.8
Lateral ankle triggerband

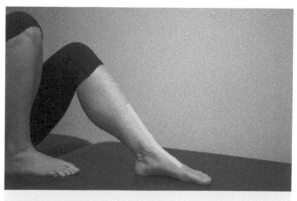

FIGURE 15.10
Anterior ankle triggerband

Achilles triggerband

Triggerbands can be found anywhere along the Achilles tendon. They are frequently seen on the medial edge, lateral edge, and through the body of the tendon (Fig. 15.11).

Ankle continuum distortions (CDs)

As stated earlier, CDs are one of the most common distortions identified in ankle injuries. Continuum technique should be applied to the areas that a patient identifies using a single finger to identify a spot of pain. Fig. 15.12 shows the most common ankle CD locations. It is critical to remember that CDs occur wherever a patient identifies them, and the practitioner must address the patient's complaint to be successful in treating the sprain.

Ankle herniated trigger points (HTPs)

While less common in the ankle, herniated trigger points can occur with ankle injuries. Generally, it is thought that soft tissue (fascia, fat, etc.) is pushed through a fascial plane and, due to tension within the plane, remains stuck in that protruding position. The patient will identify this distortion by pressing multiple fingers or their thumb into the area of pain. The practitioner will be able to palpate these distortions, and the patient will identify that the practitioner is pressing on the area of their pain. Reduction of the tissue through the fascial plane will relieve pain and restore ROM. Common locations of HTPs associated with ankle sprains are shown in Fig. 15.13.

Ankle folding distortions (FDs)

Folding distortions (FDs) in ankle sprains are common. It is imperative to be able to recognize this distortion through patient gesture and description. When FDs are identified, many techniques can be applied to recreate the necessary force and vector to treat the distortion, but it is essential to remember when treating a folding distortion that the patient should experience no pain. If a patient experiences pain during treatment of an FD, the direction of force can be reversed to address the distorted folding fascia.

There are standard techniques that every FDM practitioner should be familiar with when addressing ankle folding. Any technique that successfully unfolds or refolds the fascia can be used to address FDs.

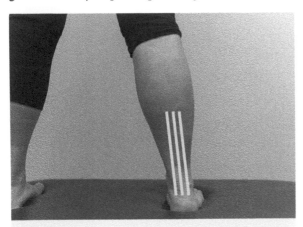

FIGURE 15.11
Achilles tendon triggerbands

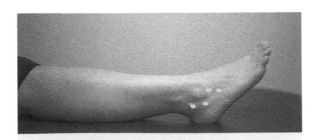

FIGURE 15.12
Common ankle continuum distortion (CD) locations

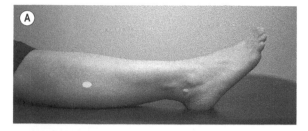

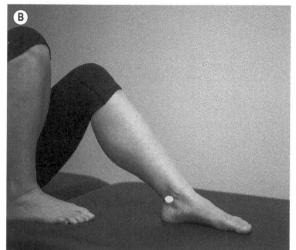

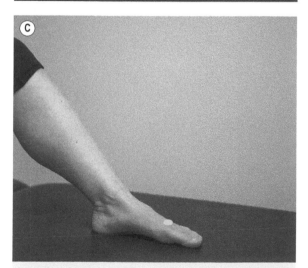

FIGURE 15.13A-C
Common locations of herniated trigger points (HTPs) associated with ankle sprains

Refolding distortions (rFDs)

To treat a refolding distortion (rFD) the refolded ankle needs to be put in the position of injury. Many variations and directions may need to be attempted to get the correct compressive force to correct this distortion. Two common methods of refolding the ankle have been taught in most courses (shown in Fig. 15.14A and B).

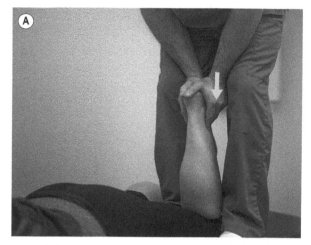

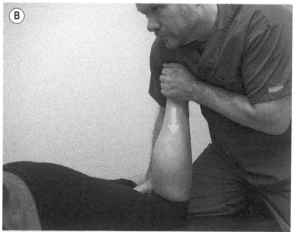

FIGURE 15.14A, B
Ankle refolding treatment

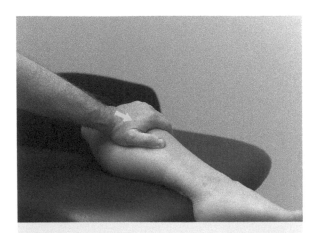

FIGURE 15.15
Interosseous membrane refolding treatment for lower extremity

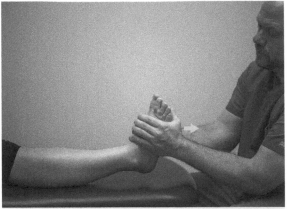

FIGURE 15.16
Ankle tug treatment for unfolding distortion (uFD) in ankle

The interosseous membrane of the lower extremity can also develop an rFD. To address this refolding, the fibula is compressed towards the tibia (Fig. 15.15).

Unfolding distortions (uFDs)

Unfolding distortions (uFDs) are treated by recreating the mechanism of injury, unfolding the fascial tissue and allowing it to return to normal physiologic position and function. There are many useful techniques to unfold the ankle. Since every injury is unique, slight variations of vector and force may be employed when using each technique.

Ankle unfolding

The straight-leg ankle thrust can be performed with two common hand grips. Traction is applied until the barrier is felt. At this point a traction thrust is applied to the ankle (Figs. 15.16 and 15.17).

Seated thrust

The ankle can be unfolded with a force applied along the tibia and out the foot while stabilizing the

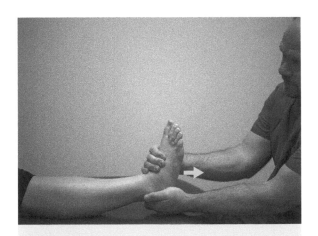

FIGURE 15.17
Ankle tug treatment for unfolding distortion (uFD) in ankle, alternate hand placement

patient's thigh against the practitioner's back. This thrust maneuver unfolds the ankle joint. Again, various vectors of treatment may need to be attempted to find the angle of force required to correct the underlying distortion (Fig. 15.18).

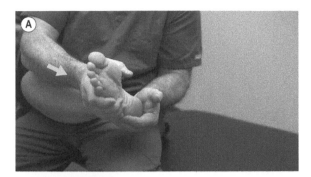

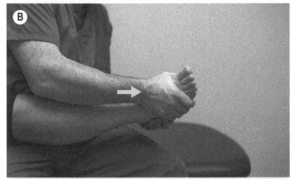

FIGURE 15.18A, B
Seated ankle thrust for unfolding distortion (uFD)

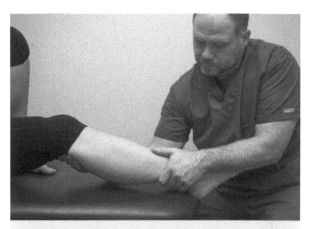

FIGURE 15.19
Forearm torque technique for unfolding treatment of ankle and interosseous membrane

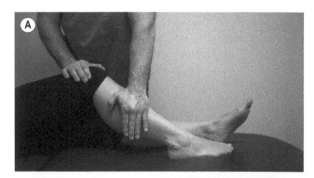

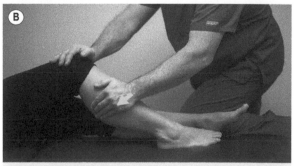

FIGURE 15.20A, B
Interosseous membrane unfolding treatment for lower extremity

Forearm torque unfolding technique

uFDs of the interosseous membrane commonly accompany inversion ankle sprains. The torque occurring in the lower leg can transmit up through the interosseous membrane between the tibia and fibula. To unfold this membrane, traction on the ankle with torque may need to be applied to correct the distortion. The forearm torque technique can be used to unfold the ankle while recreating the mechanism of injury to the interosseous septum (Fig. 15.19).

Unfolding the interosseous membrane of the lower leg may also be accomplished with a shearing force applied to the interosseous membrane that pushes the fibula away from the tibia (Fig. 15.20).

Cylinder distortions (CyDs) of the ankle

Cylinder distortions (CyDs) occur when the most superficial fascia located just beneath the skin is not able to move physiologically. Anything that restricts or inhibits the free movement of the skin and superficial fascia may cause a CyD, but the most common cause in ankle injuries is iatrogenic. Practitioners attempt to stabilize an ankle injury using a wrap, splint, or brace, which restrain the ankle, but also inhibit the normal sliding mechanism of the cylinder fascia. The formation of a CyD may contribute to edema in the sprained ankle. Patients experiencing CyDs may complain of tingling, numbness, or pain that jumps from place to place. The pain they feel may be of inexplicable intensity and may be nearly unbearable. Treatment of these distortions begins with removal of the offending restraint if one has been used. Mobilization of the skin over the superficial fascia serves to uncoil the tangled fascial coils.

Common modalities for treating CyDs in this area include manual techniques such as the squeegee and double-thumb technique (Figs. 15.21 and 15.22). Additionally, mechanical techniques can be used. A common tool used by the FDM practitioner is the cup (Fig. 15.23).

Tectonic fixations (TFs) of the ankle

Tectonic fixations (TFs) can occur between any fascial surfaces. When the fascial surfaces of the ankle are not able to slide and glide on one another, the ankle can become tectonically fixed or "frozen." TF is not typically an acute finding in ankle injuries; rather, it occurs after prolonged immobilization. The patient may have used a brace or splint for a prolonged period, or they may be limited in their range of motion due to pain and the pain they are experiencing behaves like a psychologic or behavioral splint, limiting the movement of the joint. Patients will describe the joint as being stuck and immobile.

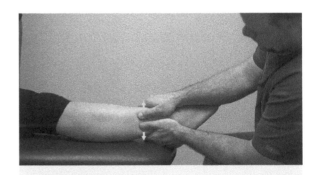

FIGURE 15.22
Double-thumb technique

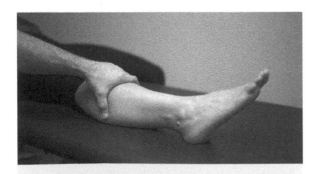

FIGURE 15.21
Squeegee technique

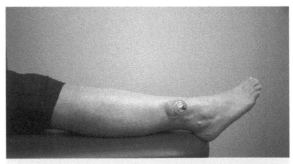

FIGURE 15.23
Cupping

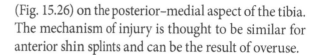

To treat this distortion, the ankle is first heated to make the fluid between the fascial layers thinner, then the ankle is mobilized in a slow, methodical pumping of the joint. The goal is to move fluid between the fascial layers, restoring the normal physiologic ability of the layers to glide and slide. Remember that TFs themselves are not considered to be painful, although they may be accompanied by painful distortions like triggerbands or CDs. In order to effectively mobilize the fascial layers, the practitioner should treat painful distortions as the patient identifies them, removing the behavioral splint and allowing the tectonic pump to move through a full ROM.

Lower leg

Shin splints

Shin splints a commonly diagnosed condition, consisting of pain along the anterior tibial spine. The fascia-bone continuum in this area can be distorted leading to the formation of CDs and these CDs are often the source of shin splint pain (Fig. 15.24). Additionally, patients may have triggerbands in the same area (Fig. 15.25).

Posterior shin splints

Posterior shin splints is similar to anterior shin splints and is often the result of CDs and triggerbands (Fig. 15.26) on the posterior–medial aspect of the tibia. The mechanism of injury is thought to be similar for anterior shin splints and can be the result of overuse.

Osgood–Schlatter disease or tibial tubercle pain

The condition known commonly as Osgood–Schlatter disease is usually associated with single spots of pain. These single spots identified by a single finger pointing to a bony location indicate CDs. Often, many CDs are present. Treating them as the patient identifies them generally provides relief of this condition. Small triggerbands have been described in this condition as well, and these should be treated using the standard technique.

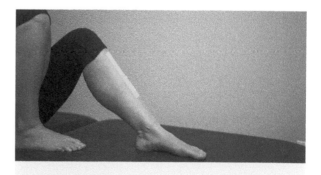

FIGURE 15.25
Anterior tibial triggerband

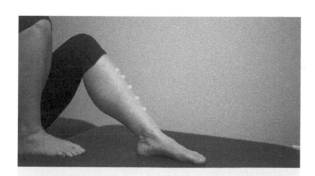

FIGURE 15.24
Common tibial continuum distortion (CD) locations

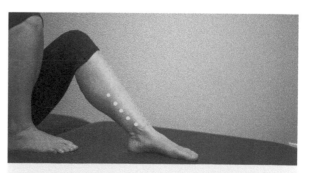

FIGURE 15.26
Common locations of posterior tibial continuum distortions (CDs)

HTPs

Lower extremity HTPs occur wherever a patient demonstrates them. Several HTPs have been named due to their prevalence:

Lateral leg HTP

This HTP can be found along the lateral aspect of the lower leg and is associated with the neurovascular bundle found there.

Peroneal nerve HTP

This HTP is commonly associated with pain around the knee and in patients with fibular head dysfunction (Fig. 15.27).

Calf HTP

The calf can develop HTPs. A high index of suspicion for deep vein thrombosis (DVT) is important when patients describe this distortion, and it is critical that the practitioner is confident that a DVT is not present before an attempt at reducing any calf HTP (Fig. 15.28).

Retrocalcaneal HTP

In patients experiencing pain in the Achilles tendon, triggerbands are common, but HTPs may also be present. The gesture associated with retrocalcaneal

HTP is a pinching of the space behind the Achilles (Figs. 15.29). Treatment involves reducing the HTP.

TFs and FDs of the lower leg
Intermuscular septal folding of the lower extremity

The intermuscular septal tissue of the lower extremity can become folded or tectonic. When an FD is present, the patient will gesture by pressing multiple fingers into the intermuscular septum

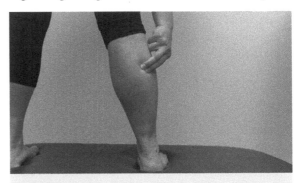

FIGURE 15.28
Gesture indicating presence and location of calf herniated trigger point (HTP)

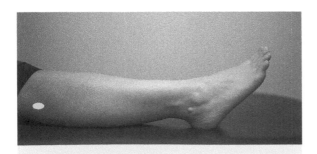

FIGURE 15.27
Peroneal nerve herniated trigger point (HTP)

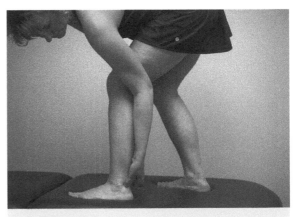

FIGURE 15.29
Gesture indicating presence and location of retrocalcaneal herniated trigger point (HTP)

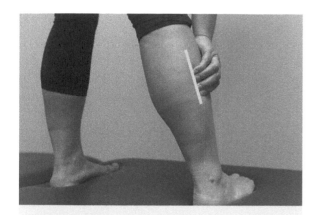

FIGURE 15.30
Gesture indicating presence and location of intermuscular septal folding distortion (FD)

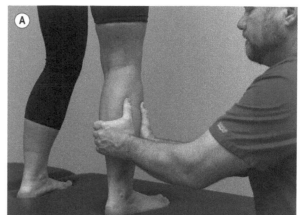

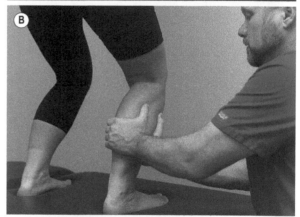

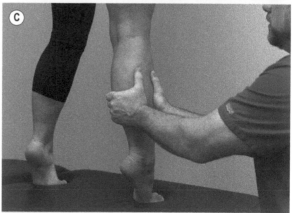

FIGURE 15.31A–C
Langton lift technique for treatment of intermuscular septal folding

(Fig. 15.30). Patients experiencing an interosseous or intermuscular septal FD may speak of pain deep in the lower leg that they are not able to locate on palpation. When the tissue is tectonic, the patient will describe a stuck feeling in the lower leg and may describe the sensation that it needs to "pop". They will experience decreased ROM but may not be experiencing pain.

Manual techniques attempting to separate the musculature with a variety of shearing forces can be applied to the lower leg. For TFs of this tissue, the technique can be employed as a tectonic pump. The Langton Lift (named after the ballet dancer Wendy [Langton] Walker, who helped develop the technique) can be used to address both of these conditions. To perform the Langton Lift, the area that is thought to be tectonic or folded is placed between the practitioner's thumbs. The practitioner places the thumbs parallel to the septum that is to be treated, then stabilizes the muscles of the lower leg while the patient proceeds through a ROM, including a squat and toe raise (Fig. 15.31).

Fibular head

The fibular head should move in a physiologic manner as a patient is walking. This motion of the fibular head is anterior–lateral and posterior–medial and if this motion is interrupted, pain is often described by the patient. All the distortions can be found with fibular head dysfunction including triggerbands, CDs, FDs and HTPs. FDs of the fibular head are a common etiology for a patient's pain.

Patients experiencing an FD of the fibular head generally gesture by grasping or holding the fibular head (Fig. 15.32). When this patient gesture is present, testing the ROM of the fibular head will often identify restriction of this area. If the fibular head is stuck posteriorly, the bone needs to be moved forward. Determining which direction of movement is painful guides the practitioner to treat the FD by moving it in the opposite direction. However, due to the location of the peroneal nerve, care must be used when assessing the ROM of the fibular head, as grasping the fibular head and putting pressure on it may cause the provider to think that movement is painful when instead pressure on the nerve is causing the pain (Fig. 15.33).

If the fibular head is stuck posteriorly and pain is not produced when it is pulled in the anterior–lateral direction, this indicates that the fibular head needs to be unfolded. Fibular head unfolding technique begins by assessing the flexion of the patient's knee. Are they able to fully flex the knee without pain? If they can perform this motion, the provider then places a hand behind the flexed knee (Fig. 15.34). The practitioner's thenar eminence or another portion of their

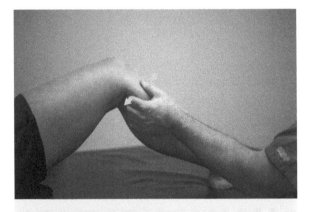

FIGURE 15.33
Motion testing of fibular head

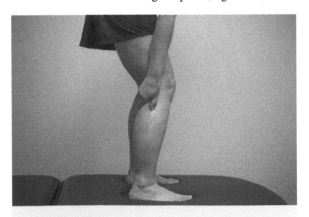

FIGURE 15.32
Gesture indicating presence and location of fibular head folding distortion (FD)

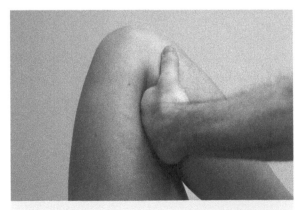

FIGURE 15.34
Hand placement for unfolding treatment of fibular head

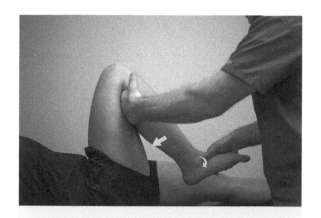

FIGURE 15.35
Unfolding treatment of fibular head set-up

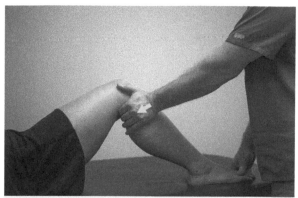

FIGURE 15.36
Fibular head refolding treatment hand placement

hand engages the fibular head. This can be assisted by introducing an external rotation of the lower leg (Fig. 15.35). When the ankle is externally rotated, the fibular head should rotate and engage the hand that is in the flexed portion of the knee. Pressure is applied to the lower leg to induce maximum flexion over the practitioner's hand, and, if this is not painful, a thrust can be applied to unfold the fibular head. Often this

treatment is associated with a "pop" as the fibular head FD is corrected. If treatment is painful, it should not be performed, and the fibular head needs to refold.

Refolding of the fibular head is achieved by forcing the fibular head more posterior–medial to the knee. This should not be painful. The fibula is thrust posteriorly behind the knee (Fig. 15.36).

Knee pain is a common complaint. All the fascial distortions can be present in the knee, and close observation of a patient's gesture, as well as careful attention to the words they use to describe their pain, guides treatment in the Fascial Distortion Model (FDM).

Knee triggerbands

Knee triggerbands occur wherever the patient indicates they are located. However, as with other regions, there are triggerbands that are frequently found in the same locations from patient to patient.

Patellar triggerbands

These can be found on either side of the patella or over the patellar tendon. The patient gesture will identify the precise location of the triggerband (Fig. 16.1A).

A U-shaped triggerband can also be found around the inferior pole of the patella. The entire triggerband can be present, or just the medial or lateral half (Fig. 16.1B).

Popliteal triggerbands

These triggerbands are found behind the knee. They can begin high in the hamstring and extend all the way down to the foot, even when the patient's gesture identifies only a small portion (Fig. 16.2).

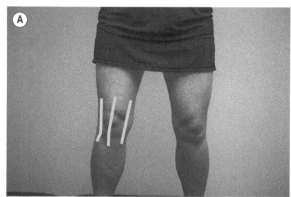

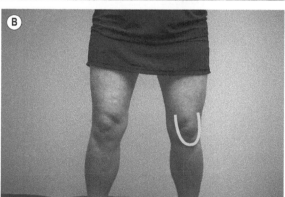

FIGURE 16.1A, B
Patellar triggerbands

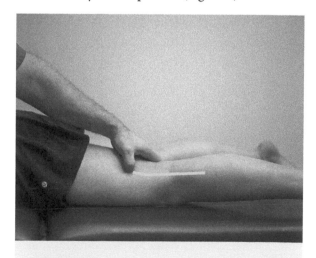

FIGURE 16.2
Popliteal triggerband

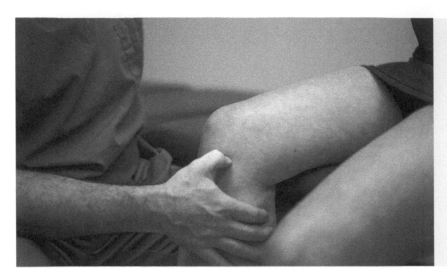

FIGURE 16.3
Location of medial joint line herniated trigger point (HTP), with example of HTP therapy

Knee herniated triggerpoints (HTPs)

A significant amount of bruising often accompanies reduction of herniated triggerpoints (HTPs) in the knee. This may be related to the neurovascular bundle as the pathway for the herniation to occur, but it also has to do with the dependent nature of the knee. The knee is generally below a patient's heart in most daily activities, so any vessel disruption below the heart will tend to accumulate more bleeding before the body repairs injury from the treatment.

Medial joint line HTPs

These pervasive distortions are identified in patients suffering from medial knee pain. Creating a gap in the medial knee can assist in the reduction of these HTPs (Fig. 16.3).

Distal thigh HTPs

HTPs in the distal portion of the anterior thigh, both lateral and medial, are a common source of knee pain. They may be related to the lateral and medial inferior genicular vascular bundles (Fig. 16.4).

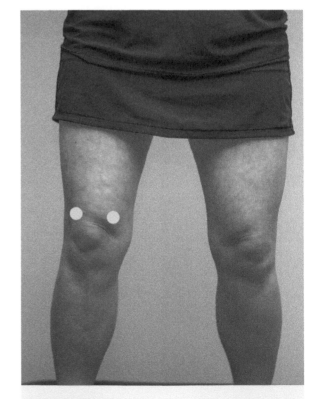

FIGURE 16.4
Distal thigh herniated trigger points (HTPs)

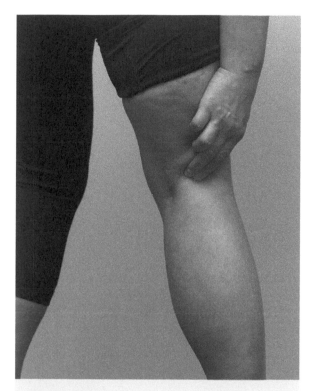

FIGURE 16.5
Patient gesture indicating presence and location of popliteal herniated trigger point (HTP)

Popliteal HTPs

Awareness of the neurovascular structures is important when treating HTPs in this area. A high index of suspicion for deep vein thrombosis (DVT) should be in the practitioner's mind when working behind the knee (Fig. 16.5).

Knee continuum distortions (CDs)

While continuum distortions (CDs) occur wherever the patient identifies them, locations for knee CDs are typically the tibial tubercle, popliteal fossa, medial joint line, lateral joint line, and the patella.

Tibial tubercle CDs

Pain along the anterior portion of the tibial tubercle is quite common and has been named Osgood–Schlatter disease. This condition can be viewed and treated as multiple CDs (Fig. 16.6).

Popliteal CDs

Most frequently located on the tibial plateau in the popliteal space, popliteal CDs are usually either medial or lateral to midline. They can be responsible

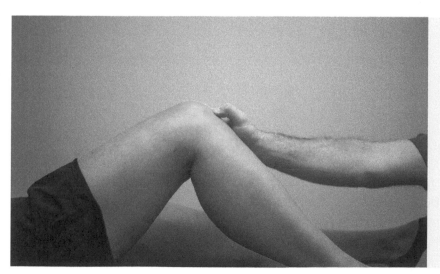

FIGURE 16.6
Continuum technique for tibial tubercle continuum distortions (CDs)

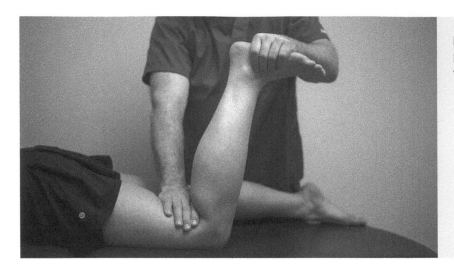

FIGURE 16.7
Hand placement for locating tibial plateau

FIGURE 16.8
Continuum technique for popliteal continuum distortion (CD)

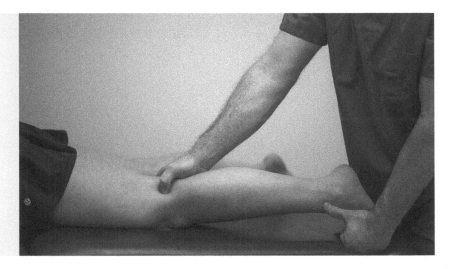

for the loss of motion in one plane, and are often found in patients describing a loss of knee flexion. When locating the tibial plateau, it is helpful to flex the knee to 90 degrees and slide a hand to the flexed point (Fig. 16.7). The hand will stop over the tibial plateau. The knee is extended back to the table, and the tibial plateau may now be palpated.

Despite their location, popliteal CDs may present with pain that refers to the anterior knee. Patients experiencing anterior knee pain should be evaluated

for this distortion if treatment following the initial pain gestures is not successful.

This distortion is also common in patients following total knee arthroplasty, and treatment may aid in recovering flexion of their knee (Fig. 16.8).

Patellar CDs

Patellar CDs are often found along the edge of the patella and even underneath it. The patella may need to be distracted or moved sideways in order

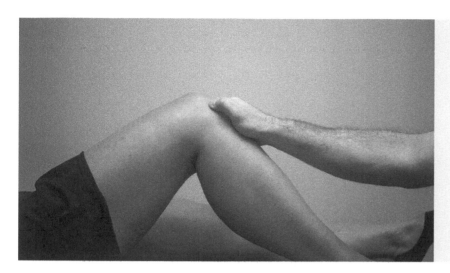

FIGURE 16.9
Continuum technique for patellar continuum distortion (CD)

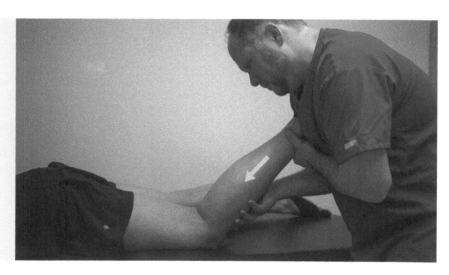

FIGURE 16.10
Refolding treatment of the knee

for the practitioner's thumb to reach the CDs (Fig. 16.9).

Knee folding distortions (FDs)
Knee refolding distortions (rFDs)

Refolding distortions (rFDs) in the knee are reported less often than rFDs in other areas of the body. This is likely due to the naturally occurring refolding mechanics taking place with each step a patient takes. Refolding treatment is often required when a more

significant force than that created by the patient's body weight is needed, or if there is an unusual twist or vector that the act of walking does not recreate (Fig. 16.10).

Knee unfolding distortions (uFDs)
Traction thrust

During this unfolding treatment, the patient lies supine with the knee extended. The practitioner grasps the leg above the ankle and applies traction to the knee. Once traction is applied, the practitioner tests

191

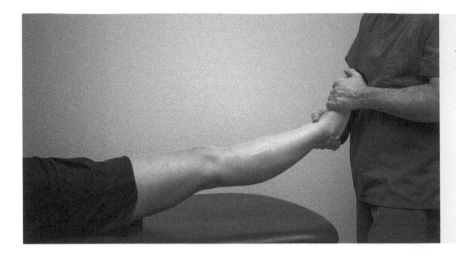

FIGURE 16.11
Traction thrust for unfolding treatment of the knee

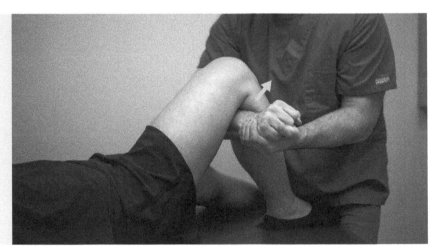

FIGURE 16.12
Forearm thrust for knee unfolding treatment

multiple vectors to find the one with the least amount of discomfort, and once established, the provides a thrust to unfold the knee joint. A rotational vector can be applied to the knee when looking for the proper set-up, and multiple thrusts may be needed to resolve the unfolding completely. This is a folding treatment and therefore, should be painless (Fig. 16.11).

Forearm thrust

This maneuver is used to unfold the knee when, in order to recreate the mechanism of injury, the tibia needs to move forward away from the femur. The technique is essentially an aggressive anterior cruciate ligament (ACL) test.

The forearm of the provider is placed behind the calf of the involved knee. Traction is applied, and the patient is asked if this is painful. If the patient reports pain in the knee, it is not the correct treatment. Proper positioning of the muscular part of the practitioner's forearm against the patient's calf prevents nerve entrapment from their grip. When a barrier is reached, and no pain is appreciated by the patient, a sharp thrust accentuating the movement is applied (Fig. 16.12).

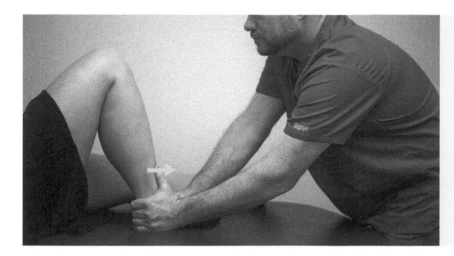

FIGURE 16.13
Whip technique, start position

FIGURE 16.14
Whip technique, end position

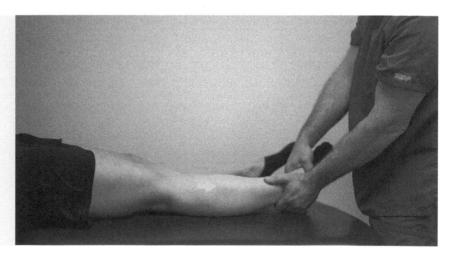

The whip technique

The whip appears to be a very aggressive technique, but it can be performed safely if the practitioner remembers that folding treatments do not hurt, and uses this maxim to guide both their set-up and treatment.

The patient lies supine with their knees flexed enough to allow their feet to rest on the treatment table. The knee is flexed as the foot is slid along the table towards the buttock, then the heel is slowly slid away from the buttock, extending the knee through its range of motion (ROM). The practitioner begins treatment with slow movements, and then, if the patient experiences no pain, increases the speed of the movements. If the maneuver is painless, the knee can be brought into extension rapidly, whipping the leg and causing the knee to unfold. The rapid, forceful extension creates a significant gapping of the knee and an unfolds the fascial matrix (Figs. 16.13 and 16.14).

Frog-leg knee technique

Just as with the frog-leg treatment used in the shoulder, the hand positions and force vectors used in this technique can be challenging to master. The goal

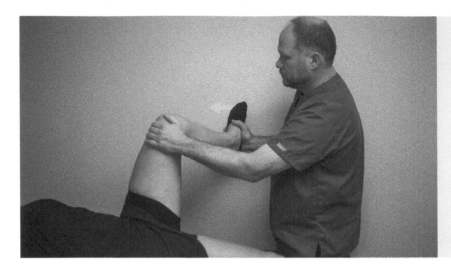

FIGURE 16.15
Frog-leg of the knee, internal rotation

FIGURE 16.16
Frog-leg of the knee, external rotation

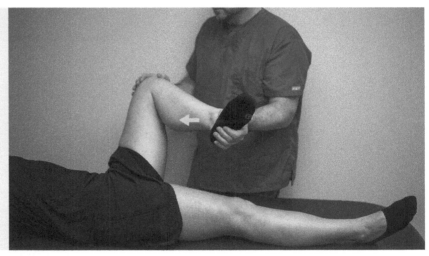

of the treatment is to unfold the misfolded fascial matrix in the knee. Misfolding is thought to occur when the knee is unfolded with a rotational force during injury.

To perform the frog-leg technique on the knee, the practitioner first flexes the patient's knee, then internally and externally rotates the leg. This rotation creates alternating medial and lateral unfolding forces in the knee. The degree of knee flexion needed to obtain the unfolding forces will vary from patient to patient: some patients require the knee to be completely flexed to feel pressure in the knee, while others require much less flexion in order to feel the unfolding. If the patient does not feel pressure in the knee, it is often an indicator that the hip is experiencing the rotational force. It is important to communicate with the patient throughout to ensure that the folding pressure is being felt correctly. Interestingly, this technique is also used to treat folding distortions in the hip (Figs. 16.15 and 16.16).

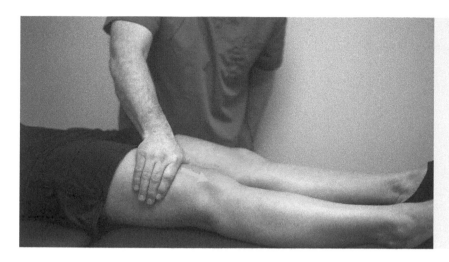

FIGURE 16.17
Squeegee technique applied to knee

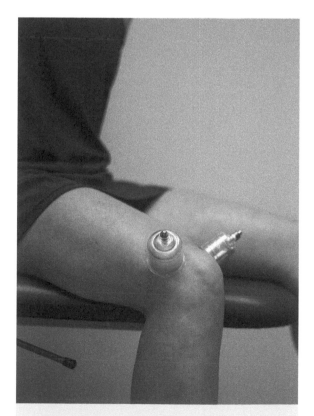

FIGURE 16.18
Common placement sites for knee cupping

Knee cylinder distortions (CyDs)

Cylinder distortions (CyDs) of the knee can be treated with both manual and non-manual techniques. It is important to remember the iatrogenic causes of CyDs in the knee. Tight clothing, braces, or compressive garments may trigger CyDs. Thrombo-embolic deterrent hose (TED hose), knee sleeves, knee braces, and post-operative boots have all been linked to CyDs in the knee.

Knee squeegee technique

Given the size of the knee relative to most practitioners' hands, the squeegee technique can be quite effective at straightening the tangled fascial coils surrounding the knee (Fig. 16.17).

Cupping with movement

This modality is quite effective for treating CyDs. The most significant complication is finding a location that the cup will remain attached while the patient goes through a ROM. Multiple cups are often utilized to treat this distortion (Fig. 16.18).

Knee tectonic fixations (TFs)

Tectonic fixation (TF) of the knee is relatively common, and is most likely the leading cause of knee replacement surgery. As with all TFs, this distortion occurs due to other distortions being present, causing pain and restricted movement, and leading to the fascial surfaces becoming sticky and tectonic.

Treatment of TF begins with heating the joint, followed by the practitioner putting the knee through motion known as the "tectonic pump". The practitioner rhythmically flexes and extends the knee, pressing and holding the knee at maximum stretch each time, to mobilize fluid in the fascial matrix. Many knee folding techniques can be used to treat TFs of the knee. Painful distortions should be treated as they are identified.

Iliotibial (IT) band

Pain in the lower extremity, thigh, and knee is often diagnosed as being the result of tension or dysfunction of the iliotibial (IT) band. Dysfunction of the IT band is commonly identified as tightness and patients are routinely prescribed stretching exercises to relieve this tightness. If stretching does not reduce the tightness, using the FDM can be very effective at improving the overall function of the IT band and lower extremity. Following the gestures and verbal description provided by a patient, the six fascial distortions can be found to impact the IT band and its function.

IT triggerbands

Tightness, pulling, and burning are classic symptoms described by patients who present with the diagnosis of IT band syndrome. This is also the definition of a triggerband. A patient gesture can direct a provider to the precise location of triggerbands that need to be treated in order to relieve symptoms of so-called IT band syndrome (Fig. 16.19).

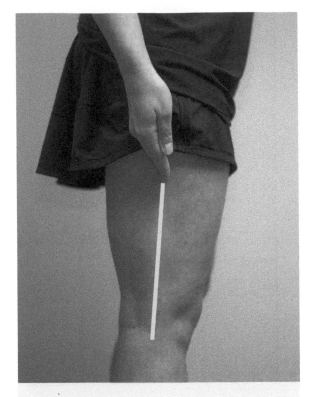

FIGURE 16.19
Gestures indicating presence and location of iliotibial (IT) triggerband

IT band HTPs

Dr Typaldos identified HTPs all over the body. In early versions of his text, he identified the thigh as a common location of this distortion, with a significant impact on the function of the IT band and therefore the lower extremity itself.

IT band HTPs are classically found in the area where the two branches of the lateral femoral cutaneous nerve pierce the IT band and continue to the surface of the skin, innervating the lateral thigh. Understanding the location of these neurovascular penetrations of the IT band can make locating the associated IT band HTPs much easier. Reduction of

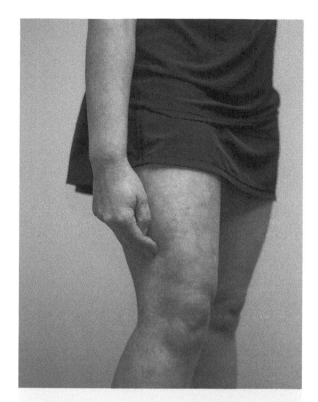

FIGURE 16.20
Gesture indicating presence and location of iliotibial
herniated trigger point (IT HTP)

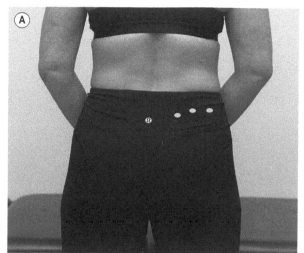

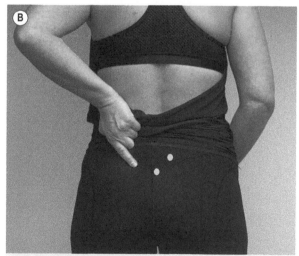

FIGURE 16.21A, B
continuum distortions (CDs) of the iliac crest and
sacral border associated with lateral thigh pain

these HTPs will often provide an immediate reduction in the tension of the IT band and dramatic symptomatic improvement for patients (Fig. 16.20).

The region of the lateral geniculate nerve marks the location of another HTP that can have an impact on the function of the IT band. When identified, treatment of this HTP can provide immediate improvement of symptoms and functionality.

IT CDs

Patients experiencing pain in the lateral thigh may have associated CDs of the iliac crest or the sacral border. Both locations can be either the cause or the result of distortions in the banded fascia of the lateral thigh (Fig. 16.21).

IT FDs

Patients diagnosed with IT band syndrome or lateral thigh pain may describe their pain as deep in the

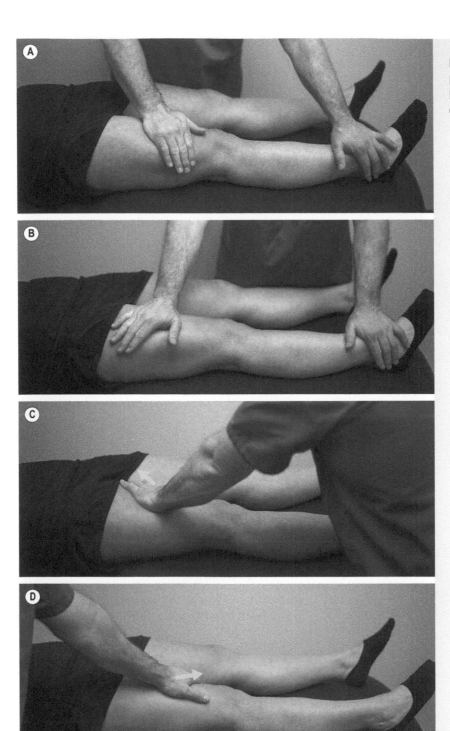

FIGURE 16.22A–D
Intermuscular septal mobilization for Iliotibial folding distortion (IT FD)

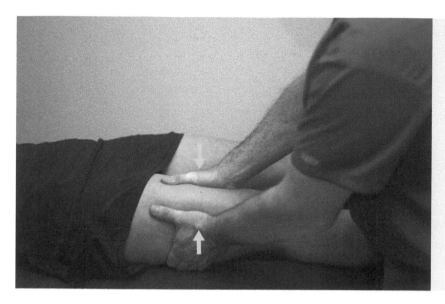

FIGURE 16.23
Intermuscular septal refolding treatment employing compression towards the femur

thigh, and may gesture with deep pressing into the lateral thigh. This deep pain cannot be palpated by the patient or the practitioner. This represents an FD of the intermuscular septum of the thigh.

Treating the folding of the intermuscular septum involves mobilizing the fascial space between two (or more) muscles. This fascial separation between the muscles needs to be moving freely, and when it is restricted or unable to move freely, patients will experience pain.

Techniques that can be used to mobilize intermuscular septal tissue require that the muscles be separated, and movement of the fascial membrane be encouraged. Manual techniques that shear the muscle from the bone at a 45-degree angle can be used, and, since this is a folding technique of the unfolding variant, the treatment should not be painful. If a patient experiences pain when the practitioner treats an FD, then either the angle of treatment is incorrect, or the diagnosis is wrong. If one angle of treatment causes pain, the practitioner should change the direction to see if this treatment is appropriate: if

unfolding the muscle from the underlying femur by pressing the tissue at a 45-degree angle to the bone causes pain, treatment can be changed to the other vectors (Fig. 16.22A–D). If all attempts to unfold this tissue cause pain, then the tissue may need to be refolded, or the diagnosis of intermuscular septal folding distortion may be incorrect (Fig. 16.23).

An additional technique named the Fairbanks Twist (named for the town in Alaska where it was first used) can be performed on the thigh. This technique involves stabilizing the musculature with the practitioner's hands on either side of the intermuscular septum that is the source of the patient's pain. Generally, the practitioner's thumbs are parallel to the septum being treated, with the intermuscular septum located between their thumbs. Care should be used to ensure the thigh is grasped with a straight-fingered grip so that the tissue is squeezed (Fig. 16.24) not pinched in a claw grip (Fig. 16.25). Once the muscles on either side of the septum are stabilized, the patient is asked to squat, mobilizing the septal tissue (Figs. 16.26 and 16.27). Alternatively, the patient can flex the knee, bringing their heel towards their buttock.

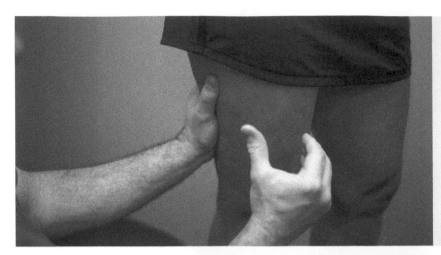

FIGURE 16.24
Fairbanks Twist hand grip.
Note the lack of curl in the
fingers.

FIGURE 16.25
Incorrect finger position for
Fairbanks Twist

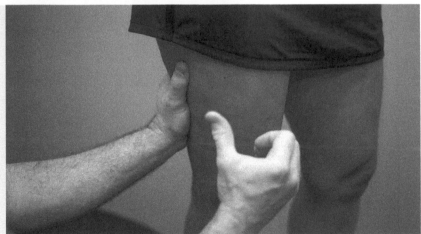

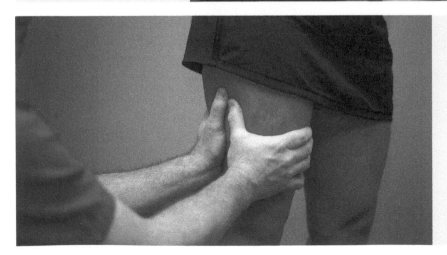

FIGURE 16.26
Hand placement for Fairbanks
Twist

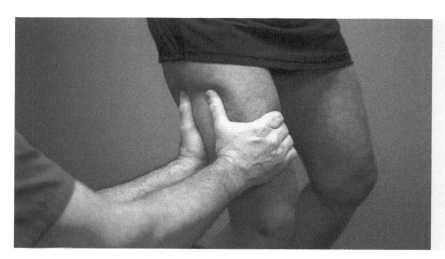

FIGURE 16.27
Patient mobilizing thigh while practitioner stabilizes muscles

IT CyDs

CyDs of the lateral thigh may be present in patients with the diagnosis of IT band syndrome. These patients describe unusual or bizarre pain, often of inexplicable intensity. Their gesture may be sweeping or squeezing the thigh if a cylinder is present. CyDs may be treated with manual or non-manual techniques.

Triggerbands of the hip

Three of the triggerbands occurring in the area of the hip are so common they have been given names. As with all triggerbands, the location is precisely where the patient gestures.

Posterior thigh triggerband

The posterior thigh triggerband begins at or near the tip of the coccyx and travels along the ipsilateral sacroiliac (SI) joint. It often follows the iliac crest and then courses down the thigh, generally passing behind the greater trochanter of the hip (Fig. 17.1).

Lateral thigh triggerband

This triggerband begins along the lateral iliac crest and travels down the lateral thigh. Often it passes over the greater trochanter of the thigh, or slightly anterior to the trochanter, and often includes portions of the iliotibial band (Fig. 17.2).

Inguinal triggerband

The inguinal triggerband is generally located between the pubic rami and the anterior superior iliac spine (ASIS). A sweeping motion across the groin is indicative of this triggerband (Fig. 17.3).

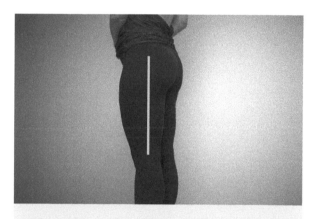

FIGURE 17.2
Lateral thigh triggerband

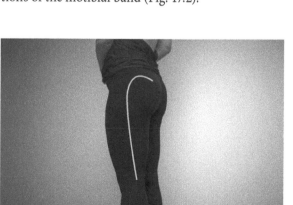

FIGURE 17.1
Posterior thigh triggerband

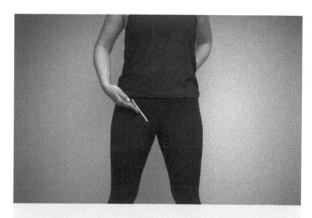

FIGURE 17.3
Inguinal triggerband

Herniated trigger points (HTPs) of the hip

Greater trochanteric HTP

Herniated trigger point (HTPs) are relatively common around the greater trochanter, or "point," of the hip (Fig. 17.4). This distortion is often found in patients previously diagnosed by traditional medical providers with greater trochanteric bursitis.

Bullseye HTP

This classic HTP is generally located over the region of the piriformis and may be associated with complaints of hip pain (Fig. 17.5).

Medial cluneal nerve HTP

There are subtle variations in location when an HTP is described over the buttock region. One of these variants is in the region of the medial cluneal nerve. The patient will gesture near the SI joint or lateral edge of the sacrum with multiple fingers (Fig. 17.6).

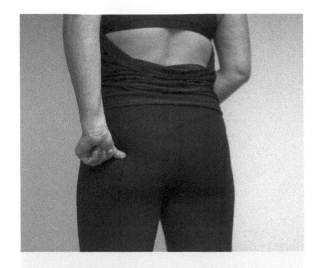

FIGURE 17.5
Bullseye herniated trigger point (HTP)

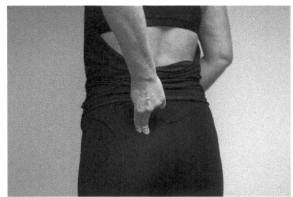

FIGURE 17.6
Medial cluneal nerve herniated trigger point (HTP)

Superior cluneal nerve HTP

Several branches of the superior cluneal nerves travel near the upper edge of the iliac crest. This location is a common location for HTPs associated with both low back and hip pain, with patients often reporting pain radiating down the lateral aspect of the leg or into the groin (Fig. 17.7).

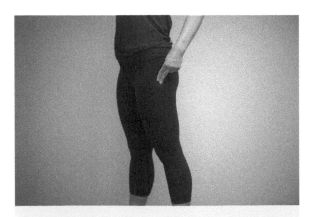

FIGURE 17.4
Greater trochanteric herniated trigger point (HTP)

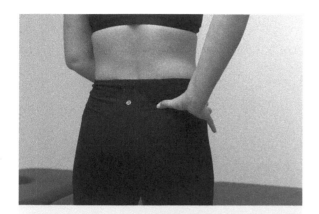

FIGURE 17.7
Superior cluneal nerve herniated trigger point (HTP)

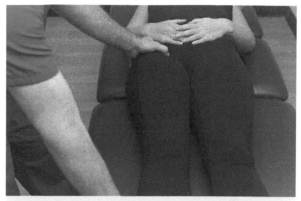

FIGURE 17.8
Herniated trigger point (HTP) therapy for inguinal HTP with patient assist

Inguinal HTP

Pain in the groin that is described with multiple fingers pressing into the inguinal region may indicate an inguinal HTP. With pain in this region, it is important to consider the diagnosis of a true inguinal hernia. If the practitioner is confident that an inguinal hernia is not present, then an inguinal HTP can be diagnosed and treated.

To treat an inguinal HTP, the femoral vessels are first palpated and located in relation to the patient's gesture, which identifies the precise location of the inguinal HTP. The patient is then instructed to place both hands on their abdomen and pull the abdominal contents in the cephalad direction. The practitioner places one thumb on the HTP, while the other hand is used to move the same side hip into flexion. Compression into the hip through the femur can also be applied. With continuous pressure on the HTP, the hip should rotate while flexed; then, when the hip is externally rotated, the leg straightens, and the hip can extend. This maneuver may simplify the reduction of the inguinal HTP. Inguinal HTPs can be treated while the patient is supine, or even in the inverted position (Figs. 17.8–17.11).

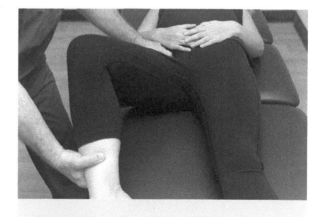

FIGURE 17.9
Herniated trigger point (HTP) therapy for inguinal HTP with external hip rotation

ASIS HTP

Close to the ASIS there is often an HTP medial or lateral to the large tendon that inserts into this bone. The patient gesture (with multiple fingers) is the same as with other HTPs. Flexion of the hip while reducing the HTP may reduce the discomfort associated with treatment.

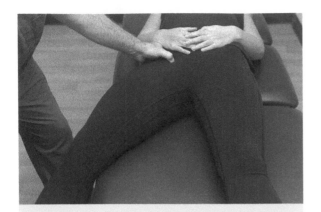

FIGURE 17.10
Hip extension following external rotation

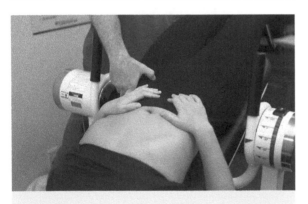

FIGURE 17.11
Herniated trigger point (HTP) therapy with inversion

Continuum distortions (CDs) of the hip

Continuum distortions (CDs) of the hip are relatively common due to the frequency of sudden-movement type injuries, such as a slip. When a patient slips and catches themselves, this can cause a CD of any bone–fascia junction.

ASIS CD

This bony landmark is a common location for single spots of pain (Fig. 17.12).

Greater trochanter CD

The bony greater trochanter is a common location for CDs.

Pubic symphysis CD

Especially common in pregnant patients, probably due to the increased mobility of the symphysis during pregnancy (Fig. 17.13).

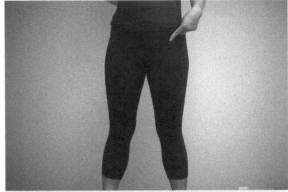

FIGURE 17.12
Anterior superior iliac spine (ASIS) continuum distortion (CD)v

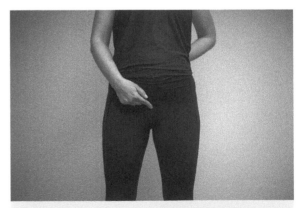

FIGURE 17.13
Pubic symphysis continuum distortion (CD)

Folding distortions (FDs) of the hip

The hip is a complex joint with many fascial planes being engaged with each movement. The fascia of the hip will often simultaneously unfold in one area and refold in another as the hip moves. This simultaneous folding and unfolding is why it is crucial to remember that treatment of FDs should not hurt. When putting a hip through a range of motion (ROM), the practitioner should be looking for the position of least discomfort.

Frog-leg technique

This technique can be utilized as both a diagnostic test and a treatment. The patient's hip is flexed, and the knee is bent. The hip is then rotated internally and externally, putting force into the joint. The tension and vector of force should be felt by the patient in the hip: if the pressure or motion is not felt in the hip, adjusting the amount of flexion of the knee can help focus the pressure into the joint being treated.

If pain is experienced while performing this maneuver, the practitioner should watch the patient's gesture to see if a triggerband, HTP, or CD needs to be addressed. Following treatment of any painful distortions, the motion is checked again, and if there is no pain, a thrust can be performed at the endpoint of the rotation (Figs. 17.14 and 17.15).

Santa Claus carry technique

This technique can be performed when an unfolding distortion (uFD) is identified in the hip, there is no pain with traction, and a significant unfolding force in the hip is required to correct the uFD identified. The practitioner places the patient's leg over their shoulder to apply force directly into the hip joint. This force can be in the form of hanging the patient from the practitioner's shoulder. A traction thrust may also be applied into the hip through the femur (Fig. 17.16).

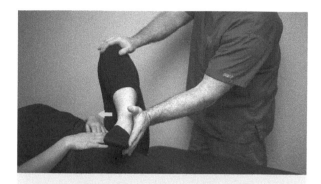

FIGURE 17.14
Frog-leg technique applied to the hip, external rotation

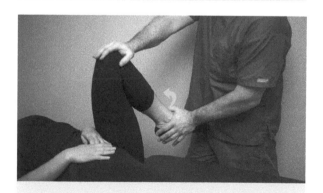

FIGURE 17.15
Frog-leg technique applied to the hip, internal rotation

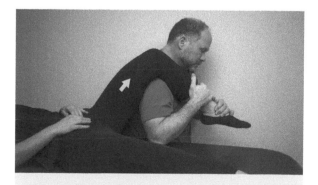

FIGURE 17.16
Santa Claus carry technique

Hip unfolding (short lever) technique

If a uFD of the hip is diagnosed, there are several methods to address this distortion. One approach is to use the patient's leg, bent at the knee, to apply a force directly into the hip joint. With the knee bent, the practitioner grasps the lower leg and thrusts through the femur, applying an unfolding force into the hip. Many different vectors of force can be used with this technique (Fig. 17.17).

Hip unfolding (long lever) technique

Treating a uFD of the hip with the knee extended, the practitioner can perform a leg tug in many planes of motion. The direction of traction causing the least amount of pain is the correct direction (Fig. 17.18).

Refolding of the hip

If there is pain when traction is applied to the hip and an FD is thought to be the diagnosis, then the force can be immediately reversed, and the joint can be compressed. This compression can be through a long or short lever (Fig. 17.19).

Thigh jar technique

When trying to mobilize the septum of the upper thigh, the muscle of the upper leg can be rotated as if the practitioner is opening or closing the lid of a jar, twisting the hamstring and the quadriceps around the femur in a clockwise or counter-clockwise fashion. Since this is an FD, this treatment should not be painful (Fig. 17.20).

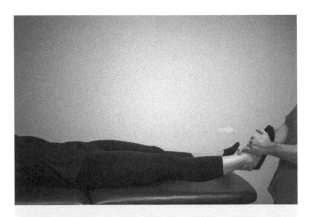

FIGURE 17.18
Hip unfolding (long lever) technique

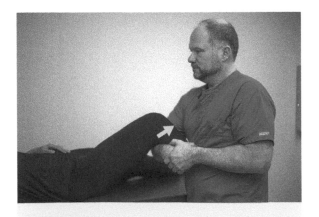

FIGURE 17.17
Hip unfolding (short lever) technique

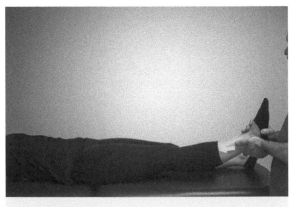

FIGURE 17.19
Hip refolding treatment

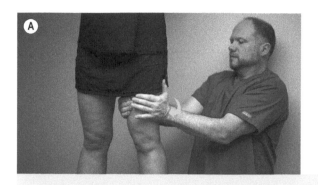

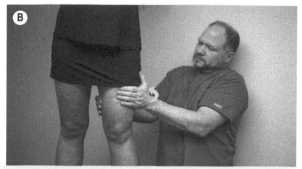

FIGURE 17.20 A,B
Thigh jar technique

Unfolding hip inversion

In stubborn uFDs of the hip, the inversion table can be used to hang the patient from one leg. While the patient is hanging, a shaking motion can be applied to encourage the folded hip tissue to unfold. Complete inversion may not be required during this treatment, and since it is an FD, there should be no pain associated with the technique (Fig. 17.21).

Cylinder distortions (CyDs) of the hip

Cylinders of the hip region often involve the lateral thigh as well as the buttock. Therefore, techniques used to treat cylinder distortions (CyDs) in this area should be able to incorporate the whole area with limited practitioner energy expenditure.

Cupping with movement

Cupping of a single area or multiple areas of the hip can cover a wide area. Cupping with movement is performed when the patient is encouraged to perform ROM maneuvers once cups are put in place (Fig. 17.22). Cupping with sliding is performed with a small amount of lubricant

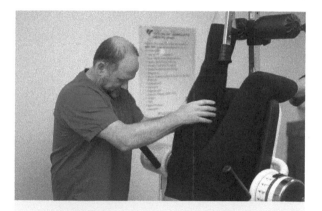

FIGURE 17.21
Inversion treatment for hip unfolding

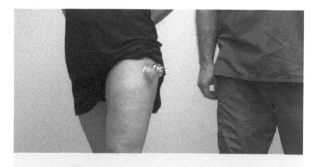

FIGURE 17.22
Cupping with movement

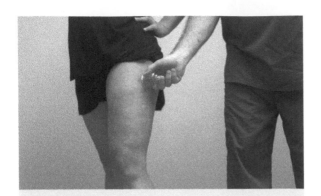

FIGURE 17.23
Cupping with sliding

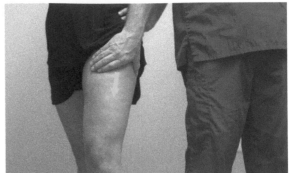

FIGURE 17.24
Squeegee technique

applied to the skin before a cup is slid across the CyD (Fig. 17.23).

Squeegee technique

The squeegee technique is performed where the hand, from thumb to index finger, contacts the skin and is slid down the leg as if the practitioner were attempting removing water from the skin surface. The goal of this treatment is to apply a constant force to the skin, pulling the tangled coil of fascia straight (Fig. 17.24).

Vacuum extractor technique

The vacuum extractor is a useful tool in the treatment of hip and lateral thigh CyDs. Traction is applied via the tool to pull the skin away from the underlying facial coils (Fig. 17.25).

Tectonic fixations (TFs) of the hip

Tectonic pump technique

When treating a tectonic fixation (TF), the first step is to heat the joint. A heat pack is applied to allow the joint fluid to warm up, reducing its viscosity. Once the joint is warm, a slow tectonic pump can be performed.

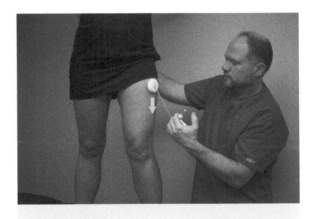

FIGURE 17.25
Vacuum extractor technique

This technique is used to induce hip motion in many planes, forcing fascial layers to separate slightly as the joint fluid is mobilized into the layers. The frog-leg of the hip can be used as a tectonic technique. Rotation of the hip is performed, and when a barrier is reached, continuous pressure is held as the fascial layers begin to slide, and the joint fluid moves between the fascial layers. A tectonic pump can also be applied through long and short lever unfolding maneuvers. The practitioner should address any other distortion the patient identifies while performing the tectonic pump.

As with any portion of the body, the Fascial Distortion Model (FDM) applied to the foot can provide powerful treatments for common ailments experienced by patients. All distortions occur wherever the patient shows them. This is just as true for the foot as with the rest of the body.

Dorsal foot pain

It is essential to observe and diagnose a patient's issues based on the gesture they demonstrate and not just the distortion one expects to see. Pain on the top of the foot can be caused by any of the distortions. The patient may display lines of pain (triggerbands), single spots of pain (continuum distortions, CDs), pain demonstrated with multiple fingers (herniated trigger points, HTPs), holding a joint (folding distortions, FDs), weird, unusual pain that is ridiculously intense (cylinder distortions, CyDs), or even a foot that feels stuck and like it needs to "pop" (tectonic fixation, TF). All these distortions occur wherever the patient shows them.

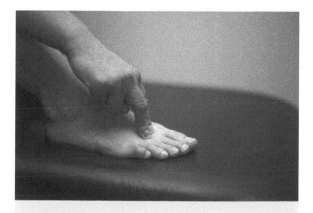

FIGURE 18.1
Dorsal foot herniated trigger point (HTP)

There are several areas on the dorsal foot that are particularly prone to developing HTPs. Across the midfoot, HTPs can form at locations associated with the neurovascular complex supplying the metatarsals. Further towards the toes, HTPs occur near the distribution of the dorsal distal branch of the peroneal nerve. This distortion is demonstrated when the patient uses multiple fingers to press the tissue on the dorsal aspect of the foot between the toes (Fig. 18.1).

Plantar foot pain

The condition of plantar fasciitis should, in many cases, be reclassified as plantar foot pain. While almost all pain that patients demonstrate on the bottom of their foot may be diagnosed by traditional medicine as plantar fasciitis, not all pain on the plantar surface is secondary to inflammation. It is important to watch and listen to the patient's presentation. Often, the patient will demonstrate a distortion that explains the pain in the FDM.

Lines of pain that feel as though they are pulling and burning on the bottom of the foot are very typical presentations for plantar foot pain. These lines of pain often begin near the heel and radiate towards the toes. Patients will describe tightness, pulling, and burning, while demonstrating the standard gesture at the location of the triggerband (Figs. 18.2 and 18.3).

In addition, two superficial cutaneous nerve bundles are found on the plantar surface of the foot. These two areas may be responsible for some cases of plantar foot pain where the patient demonstrates or gestures to the pain with multiple fingers.

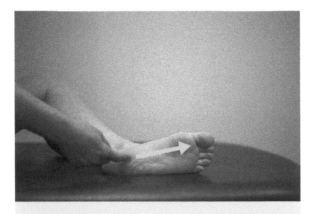

FIGURE 18.2
Plantar triggerband

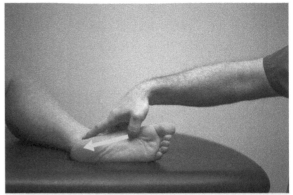

FIGURE 18.4
Triggerband technique for plantar triggerband

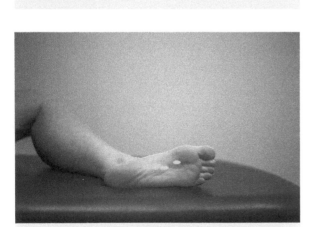

FIGURE 18.3
Common locations for plantar herniated trigger point (HTP)

Palpation and reduction of this plantar HTP can be very effective at reducing the plantar fascia pain (Fig. 18.4).

CDs on the plantar surface of the foot occur wherever the patient demonstrates them. The heel is a very common location for CDs in patients describing plantar foot pain.

Bunion

In patients experiencing pain from a bunion, FDM can help reduce the pain they are experiencing as well as improve function. The patients will demonstrate through gesture and description where they are experiencing pain. When the distortions are addressed, the patient can get significant relief of the pain associated with a bunion. In most cases, the bunion will remain, but the pain is much reduced or eliminated. It is important to follow the patient's lead and allow them to guide the practitioner in what needs to be treated. It is common for patients with a painful bunion to demonstrate triggerbands (Fig. 18.5), CDs, and FDs (Fig. 18.6).

Morton's neuroma

Morton's neuroma is frequently diagnosed when a patient presents with pain – often described by the patient as a burning pain – between their toes. Patients rarely receive imaging confirming the diagnosis of a neuroma, and even if the diagnosis is confirmed with imaging, treating fascial distortions can provide significant pain relief. Any or all of

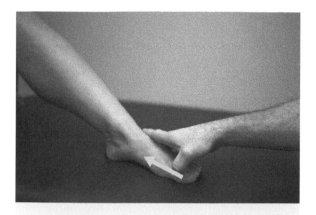

FIGURE 18.5
Triggerband technique for triggerbands identified over a bunion

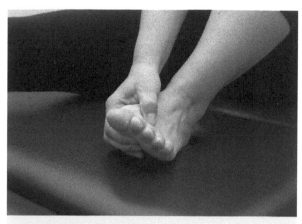

FIGURE 18.7
Morton's neuroma

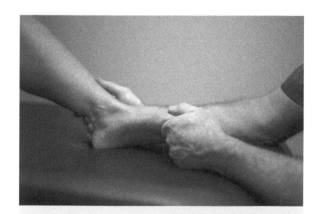

FIGURE 18.6
Refolding treatment for refolding distortion in the first toe

the distortions may be found when a patient presents with the diagnosis of a neuroma, but those most often associated with this condition include triggerbands, CDs, and FDs of the metatarsal pad, the interosseous membrane between the toes, and of the joints of the toes (Fig. 18.7).

Ledderhose disease

This condition is similar in presentation to Dupuytren's contracture of the hands (see p. 137) but when it presents in the feet, it is called Ledderhose disease. It is thought that the same pathophysiologic process occurs on the plantar surface of the feet that occurs in the palmar surface of the hands, and, as with Dupuytren's, treating Ledderhose in the FDM can provide significant symptomatic relief as well as appearing to slow the progression of the condition. Commonly the patient will identify triggerbands, HTPs, CDs, FDs, and TF of the tissues in the plantar surface of the foot (Fig. 18.8).

Achilles pain

Achilles pain, either in the tendon or at the insertion point of the tendon, is often attributed to an inflammatory condition. While this can be the cause in some cases, observing the patient's gesture and listening to their description of their pain can lead to a diagnosis of a fascial distortion. Treatment in the

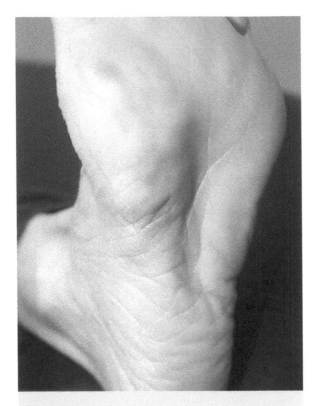

FIGURE 18.8
Ledderhose disease

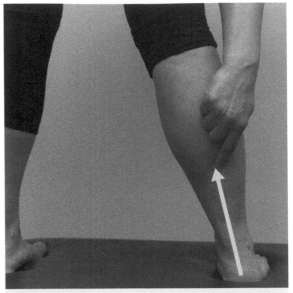

FIGURE 18.9
Achilles tendon triggerbands

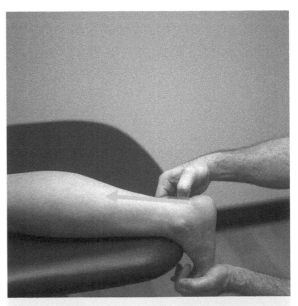

FIGURE 18.10
Triggerband technique for Achilles triggerband

FDM can provide rapid pain reduction and improvement in range of motion (ROM) and function. Swollen and tender Achilles tendons may be associated with triggerbands of the tendon itself or of the soft tissue around the tendon. This may represent a collection of triggerbands (Fig. 18.9). Treatment leads to a rapid reduction in the size of the tendon swelling, as well as decreased pain (Fig. 18.10).

In patients experiencing pain in the Achilles tendon, the insertion onto the calcaneus is often described as the location of the pain. A single finger pointing to the source of the pain is consistent with the diagnosis of a CD. CDs may be found anywhere the fascial tissue inserts into the calcaneus (Fig. 18.11).

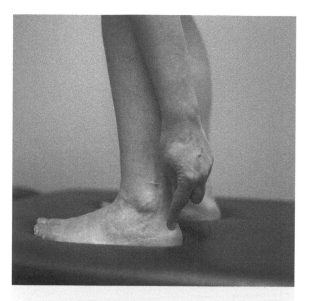

FIGURE 18.11
Patient gesture indicating the presence and location of a continuum distortion (CD)

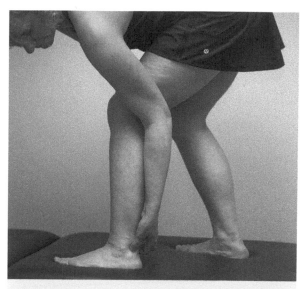

FIGURE 18.12
Patient gesture indicating the presence and location of retrocalcaneal herniated trigger point (HTP)

Pinching the space behind the Achilles tendon appears to be associated with an HTP in the area of the retrocalcaneal bursa. This HTP has been named the retrocalcaneal HTP. The same plateau of the calcaneus is also the location of CDs in some patients experiencing pain in the Achilles tendon (Fig. 18.12).

Metatarsalgia

Pain at the heads of the metatarsals can occur for many different reasons. When viewed through the lens of FDM, all the distortions can contribute to the cause of pain in this region. There is thought to be shock-absorbing fascia in the metatarsal pads, the distortion of which can be the etiology of FDs in the area (similar to that described in the heel pain section below). Other distortions can also be identified and should be treated, including triggerbands, HTPs, and CDs (Fig. 18.13).

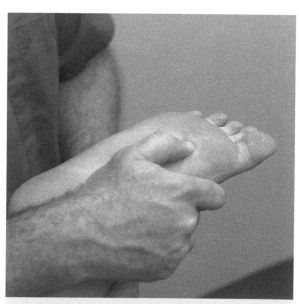

FIGURE 18.13
Treating distortions in the metatarsal pads

Heel pain

Heel pain is a common condition. Viewed through the FDM, watching for the classic gestures as well as listening to the patient's description of pain can lead to the identification of distortions that, when treated, provide significant pain relief and improved function. CDs of the calcaneus and calcaneal spur are found in patients that describe their pain with a single finger pointing to the spot of pain (Fig. 18.14). Some patients will describe a line of pain around or through the heel, consistent with a triggerband. When multiple fingers are pressed into the heel pad, an HTP has been identified (Fig. 18.15).

At times, the patient may grasp the heel with the thumb and index finger in a C-shape surrounding the heel (Fig. 18.16). This gesture is interesting and somewhat unique to the heel. In the FDM, this could be a line of pain, representing a triggerband.

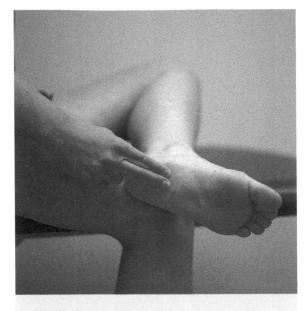

FIGURE 18.15
Calcaneal herniated trigger point (HTP)

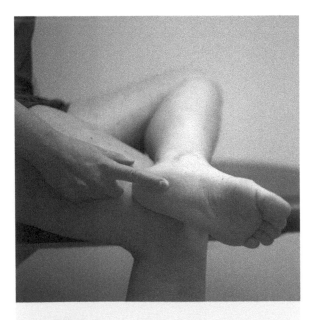

FIGURE 18.14
Calcaneal continuum distortion (CD)

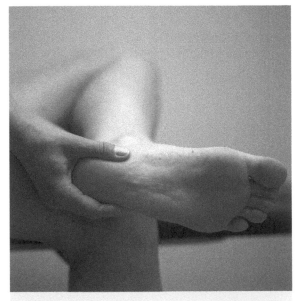

FIGURE 18.16
"C-shape" gesture at the heel

If this line was painful along its entire course, then that would represent the most likely diagnosis, and would need to be treated. However, if the line is not painful, then this gesture could represent an FD of the heel pad. Recall that FDs are associated with the gesture where the patient holds the folded tissue and

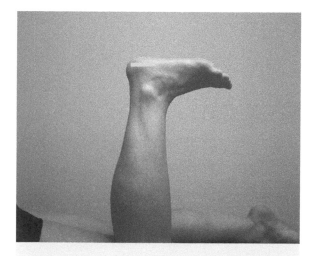

FIGURE 18.17
Location of heel triggerband and folding distortions (FDs)

complains of pain deep inside the joint. While the heel pad and its function may not be considered by most to be a joint, the heel is comprised of folding fascia that refolds and unfolds (Fig. 18.17). When tissue moves in a folding fashion, FDs can occur, and when a heel pad is overly compressed, a refolding distortion (rFD) of the heel can occur. This would be treated by refolding or compressing the heel.

Two different techniques can be used to refold the heel (see Figs. 18.18 and 18.19). If compression of the heel is painful, then an unfolding distortion (uFD) may be present, and this distortion can be treated by unfolding the heel pad (Fig. 18.20).

The folding mechanism of the heel has been treated by treating the line described by the patient as the folding tissue (Fig. 18.17). It has been found that when a force is placed directly onto the heel pad, the tissue in this line expands or unfolds and it is also thought that with enough force, herniated trigger points (HTPs) can form in this space. When a practitioner is presented with a patient experiencing pain in the heel, the practitioner can palpate the heel, feeling for firm areas on the surface of the

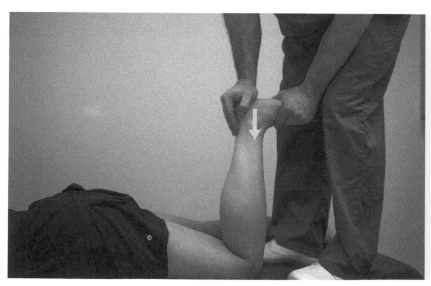

FIGURE 18.18
Refolding the heel pad

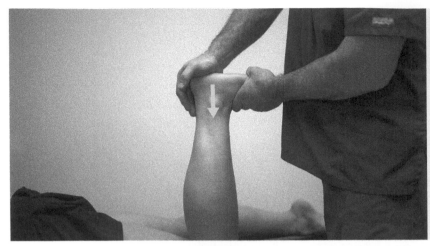

FIGURE 18.19
Refolding the heel pad, alternate position

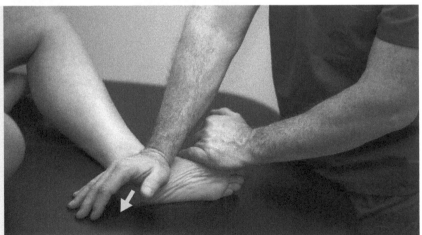

FIGURE 18.20
Unfolding the heel pad

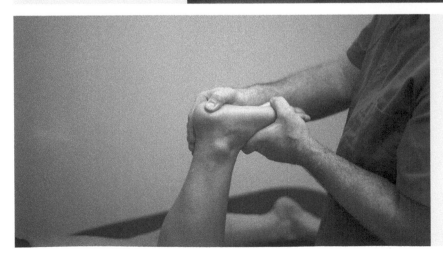

FIGURE 18.21
Palpating for firm areas in the heel

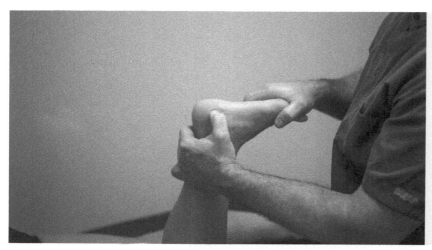

FIGURE 18.22
Treatment of heel pad distortions from a lateral approach, "tucking" pleats back into the fascia

FIGURE 18.23
Reassessing firm areas in the heel

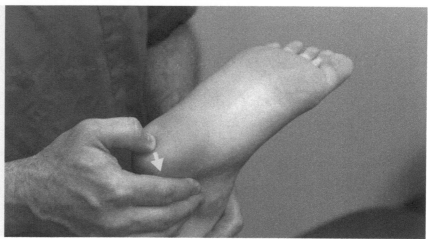

heel (Fig. 18.21). These areas feel as if the heel has lost padding, and the patient is walking on a much firmer part of the heel. When the line is addressed from the side by treating either the HTPs (painful to treat) or FDs (not painful to treat) the heel pad rapidly regains compressibility and the sensation of firmness upon compression often resolves. The treatment for either of these conditions is to press the tissue back into the heel along the line described by the patient (Fig. 18.22). It may be helpful for the practitioner to visualize "tucking" the pleats of fascia back into the folding fascia.

Following the treatment of the heel "joint line," the plantar surface of the heel is reassessed, and any remaining firm areas can be treated again (Fig. 18.23).

What is inversion treatment, and what does it mean in the Fascial Distortion Model (FDM)?

When treating patients in the FDM, Dr Typaldos encountered some truly stubborn unfolding distortions (uFDs). Even though he was confident that the pain these patients were experiencing fit within the model, their uFDs were not responding to treatment, and consequently, he felt that traditional tools and techniques were not adequate. Dr Typaldos developed the idea of using inversion tables, which take advantage of gravity and body weight to unfold the tissue in the spine and other joints by supporting patients in an upside down position.

With folding distortions (FDs), it is believed that the force of refolding or unfolding treatment needs to be the same as that which caused the initial folding injury. The spine can be visualized as a large spring that functions as a shock absorber. As with other shock absorbers, the spine is subjected to compression and distraction forces in excess of normal. These forces are in excess of the force a practitioner can apply using basic manual techniques. Recall that tensegrity dictates that no two bones ever want to come in contact. The bones of the spine are continually trying to maintain an equilibrium, repelled from the vertebra above and below through the tensegrity system maintained by ligaments, muscles, and tendons. Maintaining this separation is critical for the normal physiologic function of the spine and all joints.

If the spine is unfolded, a portion of the spine has been lengthened or distracted and a distortion in the fascial matrix has occurred. The distorted matrix will not allow these vertebrae to return to their normal placement. When there is an alteration of the folding

fascia of the spine, the shock-absorbing mechanism within the folding fascia is also lost. When treating a uFD, Dr Typaldos believed that hanging a person upside down, using their body weight to assist in the unfolding of the spine, could be effective, but testing such treatments was time-consuming and required equipment he did not have in his office. He asked Marjorie Kasten, PT, to develop inversion treatments consistent with the FDM. Marjorie Kasten was committed to treating these distortions, in part because she had experienced them herself. She has compiled some thoughts on her work in the text titled *Which Way is Up When You Are Upside Down?* (Kasten, 2010).

FDs of the spine should be suspected when the patient places a hand over the center of their back, as if they were trying to hold their spine, and/or complains of pain deep in the spine that they cannot touch (Fig. 19.1). The patient may say that they have

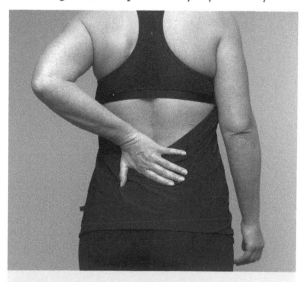

FIGURE 19.1
Spinal folding body language

"always had [the pain]" or that it has been there for a long time. Pain that changes with the weather is also attributed to FDs. Pain associated with FDs also improves or worsens when lying down or standing, depending on the type of FD present.

Inversion tables and techniques

There are two types of inversion tables: extension tables, and flexion tables. When using extension tables, the patient hangs from their feet or ankles. They are referred to in the FDM as an extension table because the spine is in the extended position (Fig. 19.2). The second type of table is referred to as a flexion table because the patient hangs from their waist with the lumbar spine in a flexed position (Fig. 19.3). Inversion tables can be used to recreate the position of injury when a folding distortion occurred, if it is known. For example, the patient wearing a seatbelt during a car accident may benefit from the use of the flexion table. Inversion treatment can be used to treat stubborn, long-standing, or persistent folding injuries of the spine.

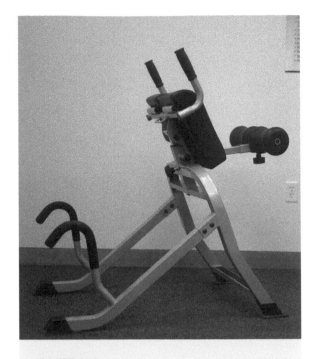

FIGURE 19.3
Flexion inversion table

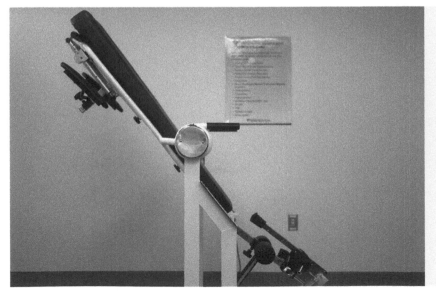

FIGURE 19.2
Extension inversion table

Using an extension inversion table

When treating a uFD in the back on an extension table, the patient hangs from their feet or ankles. The use of boots with a hook that attaches to the inversion table can reduce the amount of discomfort a patient feels in their ankles and feet. Once the patient is on the table, the table is placed horizontally with the patient face down (some styles of inversion boots will not permit this) (Fig. 19.4) or face up (Fig. 19.5). The benefit of the patient being prone on the inversion table is that the practitioner has access to the patient's back during the inversion treatment, and that inverting in this position is a more physiologic motion and so may

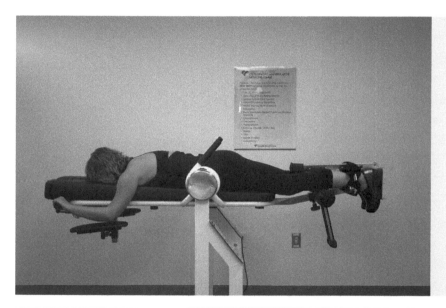

FIGURE 19.4
Extension inversion table patient, prone

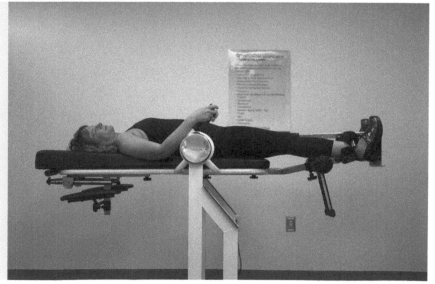

FIGURE 19.5
Extension inversion table patient, supine

be better tolerated, since it is common for patients to bend forward at the waist. In addition, some patients experience anxiety when tipped backward on the inversion table, and for these patients, placing them prone on the table may reduce the anxiety they are experiencing and allow inversion to be used.

Remember when treating folding distortions, if there is pain present, then this is not the correct treatment. Inversion should only be used with patients who think it would feel good or who feel relief while inverted.

Once a patient is inverted, they can unfold at many different angles on the table (Fig. 19.6). Complete inversion, hanging free by the feet or ankles, is not always required for a successful treatment (Fig. 19.7). Occasionally, when a patient is hanging free on the table, even more force is required to unfold the spine. This can be added by the practitioner as long as the extra force feels "right" and does not cause pain (Figs. 19.8 and 19.9). In some

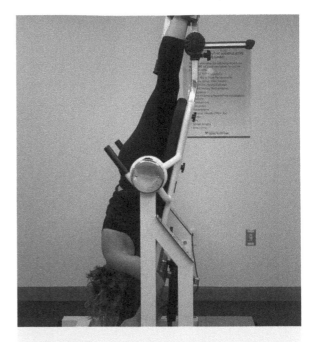

FIGURE 19.6
Full extension inversion, prone

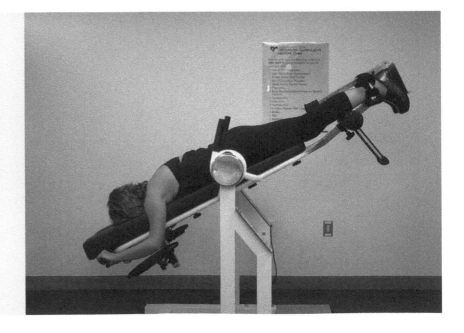

FIGURE 19.7
Extension inversion, prone, less than vertical

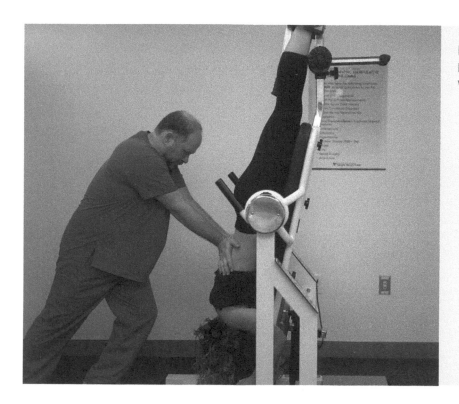

FIGURE 19.8
Extension inversion, prone, with additional force

FIGURE 19.9
Extension inversion, prone, additional force, seated

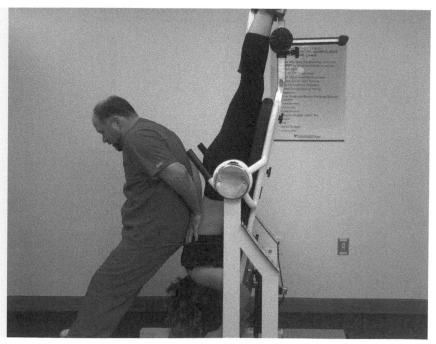

instances, when the patient is inverted, gently shaking the person can assist with further unfolding of the spine (Fig. 19.10). Any additional distortion identified while the patient is inverted can be treated while they are in that position. For example, a triggerband, herniated triggerpoint (HTP), or continuum distortion (CD) can be treated while the patient is inverted (Figs. 19.11 and 19.12). The plunger can be

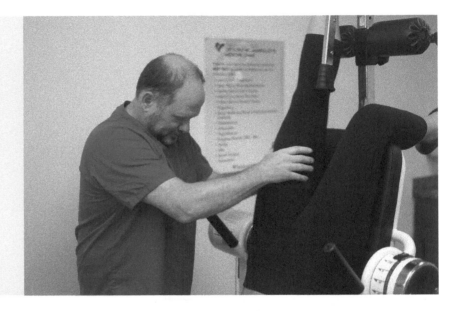

FIGURE 19.10
Extended inversion, prone – shaking treatment

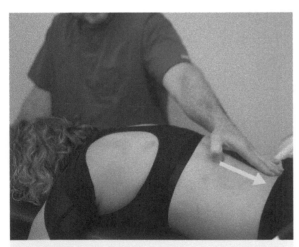

FIGURE 19.11
Extended inversion treatment of other distortion while inverted – triggerband

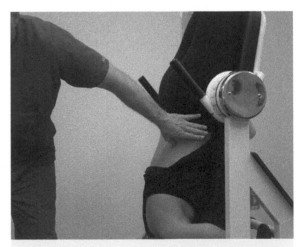

FIGURE 19.12
Extended inversion treatment of other distortion while inverted – herniated triggerpoint (HTP)

used while a patient is inverted to pull tangled cylindrical fascia from between the vertebra as well as to shake loose stubborn folding distortions in the spine (Fig. 19.13). Spinal FDs can be multi-directional, and the addition of a rotational force in the direction of decreased pain, or that "feels right", can be used to provide an additional vector of treatment (Fig. 19.14).

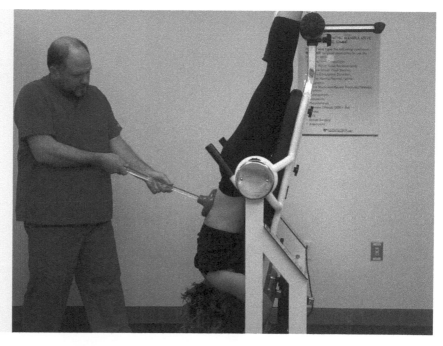

FIGURE 19.13
Extended inversion – cylinder treatment

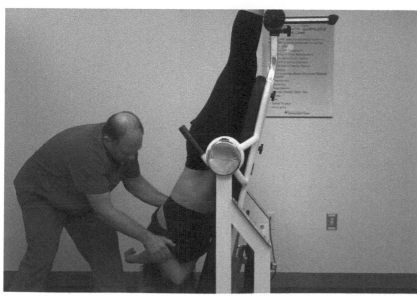

FIGURE 19.14
Extended inversion with rotation

If a joint or body region can be unfolded, the same area can be refolded. The complementary action of extended inversion is axial compression. This can be performed with direct axial compression of the spine. Generally, to treat a refolding distortion (rFD) of the thoracic and lumbar spine, the compression force is generated by the practitioner pushing straight down onto the shoulders (Fig. 19.15). As the compressive force is increased, the patient can be rotated to find the position of most comfort. The spine can be felt compressing and decompressing when the tissue is refolding correctly. Once the spine is fully compressed, the sensation that a patient feels when the compression is released can be a valuable diagnostic clue to the practitioner. If the spine springs back when released, this is considered a healthy and normal response. If there is a slow rise of the spine or the spine catches as it returns to the neutral, uncompressed position, this is considered less healthy, and it is likely that there are additional distortions present, preventing the normal function of the spine fascial matrix.

Using a peanut ball

If a patient receives significant relief with inversion, they may receive similar relief using a peanut ball at home (Fig. 19.16). The peanut ball can be more effective than a traditional exercise ball for home extension treatment because its shape is more stable than a spherical exercise ball, requiring less activation of the core muscles while a patient is relaxing on the peanut. Home extension exercises with the peanut ball can bring additional relief to the uFDs between office visits (Figs. 19.17 and 19.18). When using the peanut

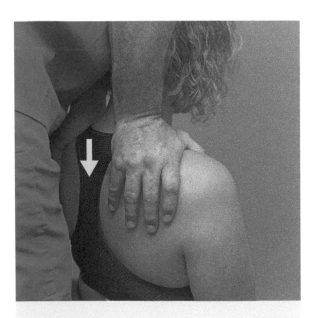

FIGURE 19.15
Axial spinal refolding

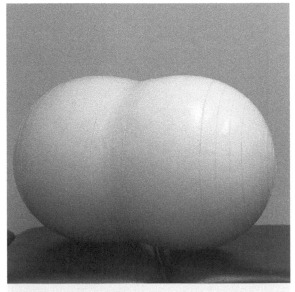

FIGURE 19.16
The peanut ball

ball at home, it is important for the patient to understand they are treating an FD, and as a rule, the maneuvers should feel good. When finishing the home stretching program, it is best if the patient rolls to a prone position on the ball before getting up (Fig. 19.19).

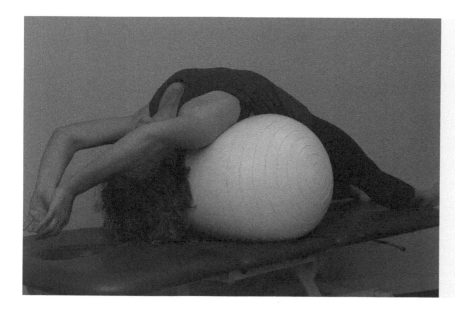

FIGURE 19.17
Peanut ball – extension

FIGURE 19.18
Peanut ball – side bending

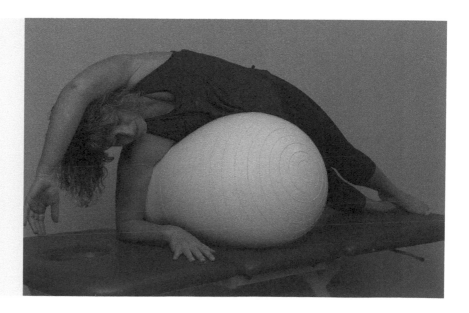

The peanut ball can also be utilized in the clinical setting. The provider can use the ball to encourage unfolding and refolding of the patient's ribs in a side-lying position. The side of the patient that is up (away from the ball) is unfolding, while the side against the ball is refolding. This treatment also places these same forces on to the vertebral segments of the spine (Fig. 19.20). Another technique called paravertebral

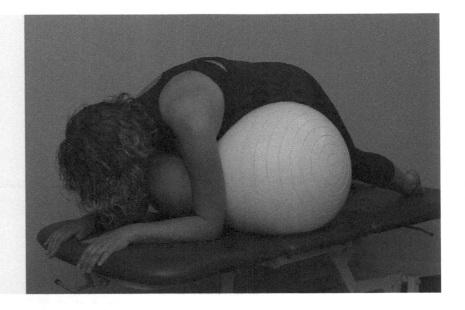

FIGURE 19.19
Peanut ball – proper dismount

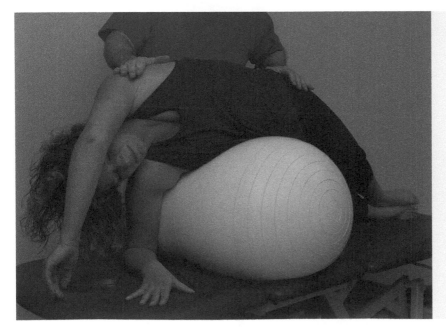

FIGURE 19.20
Peanut ball – rib unfolding and refolding

unfolding can be used to create an unfolding force in the spine (Fig. 19.21). The peanut ball can also be used to accentuate the flexion of the thoracic spine, assisting the treatment of distortions found between the ribs, including triggerbands, HTPs, and CDs (Fig. 19.22).

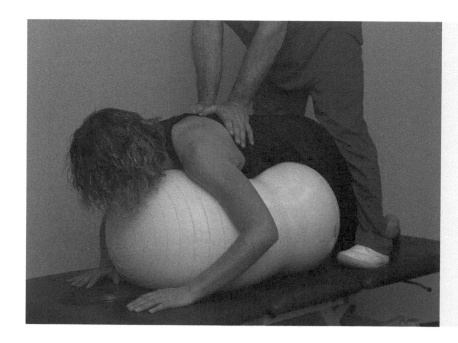

FIGURE 19.21
Paravertebral unfolding

FIGURE 19.22
Peanut ball – thoracic flexion for treatment between ribs

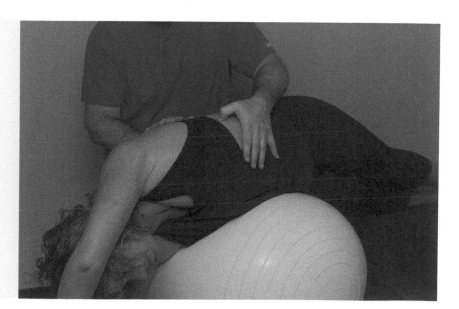

Using a flexion table

The flexion inversion table provides access to the back as well as the pelvic floor. Distortions in these areas can be addressed while the patient is hanging inverted. The flexion inversion table is especially helpful in treating patients who are experiencing spinal stenosis (Fig. 19.23). The flexion of the lumbar spine opens the foramina, creating more space for the nerves. Treatments similar to those performed on the extended inversion table are possible on the flexed inversion table (Figs. 19.24, 19.25, and 19.26).

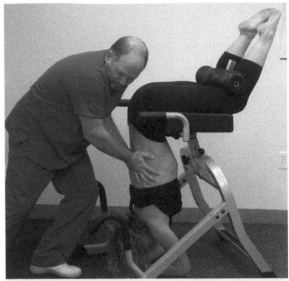

FIGURE 19.24
Flexion inversion with extra force

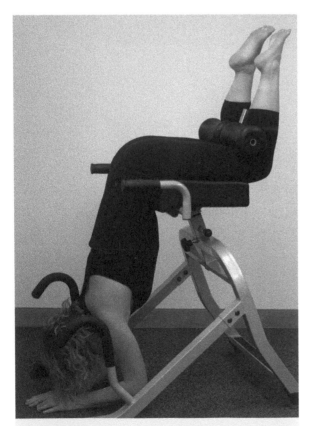

FIGURE 19.23
Flexion inversion

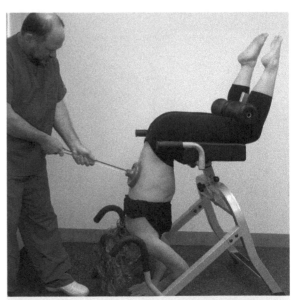

FIGURE 19.25
Flexion inversion with plunger

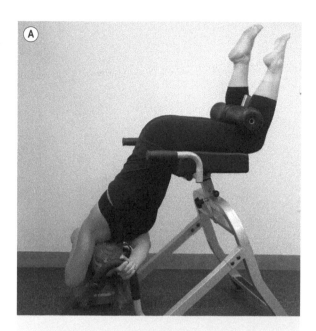

FIGURE 19.26A
Flexion inversion with rotation

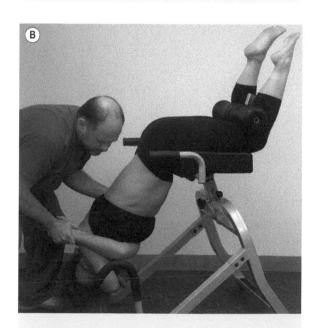

FIGURE 19.26B
Flexion inversion with rotation

Contraindications for inversion

There are many contraindications to inversion treatment to consider before inverting a patient (Box 19.1). The primary contraindications are a history of pain on inversion and the patient's sense that inversion would not feel good. If they experience pain while inverted, the patient should be evaluated for any of the painful distortions as the cause, and whether they have an rFD at the area of pain. It is possible to have a combination of unfolding and refolding in an area. These are complex treatments and require a thorough understanding of the folding and unfolding aspects of the FDM to achieve adequate relief.

Box 19.1 Inversion contraindications

Patients who have the following conditions **may not** be good candidates to use the inversion table:

- Use of anti-coagulants
- Total hip or knee replacements
- Severe spinal cord trauma
- Heart/circulatory disorders
- Hiatal hernia/ventral hernia
- Pregnancy
- Bone weakness/recent fractures/skeletal implants
- Osteoporosis
- Glaucoma
- Hypertension
- Extreme obesity (300+ lbs)
- Stroke
- TIAs
- Spinal surgery
- Aneurysms

REFERENCES AND BIBLIOGRAPHY

Adstrum, S., Hedley, G., Schleip, R., Stecco, C., Yucesoy, C.A. (2017). Defining the fascial system. *Journal of Bodywork & Movement Therapies.* (21)1, pp. 173–7. Available at: doi: 10.1016/j.jbmt.2016.11.003 [Accessed 30 Mar, 2020].

Anon. (2019). Burn-out an "occupational phenomenon": International Classification of Diseases. *World Health Organization.* Available at: https://www.who.int/mental_health/evidence/burn-out/en/ [Accessed 30 Mar, 2020].

Bachman, L.M., Kolb, E., Koller, M., Steurer, J. and ter Riet, G. (2003). Accuracy of Ottawa ankle rules to exclude fractures of the ankle and mid-foot: systematic review. *BMJ*, 327(7405). Available at: https://doi.org/10.1136/bmj.326.7386.417 [Accessed 30 Mar, 2020].

Beard, G.M. (1869). Neurasthenia, or Nervous Exhaustion. *The Boston Medical and Surgical Journal,* 80(13), pp. 217–21.

Chou, R., Fu, R., Carrino, J. and Deyo, R. (2009). Imaging strategies for low-back pain: systematic review and meta-analysis. *The Lancet,* 373(9662), pp. 463–72. Available at: https://doi.org/10.1016/S0140-6736(09)60172-0 [Accessed 30 Mar, 2020].

Cole J. and Oppenheimer A. (Hrsg.) (2005) Living without Touch and Proprioception. In: *The congress papers: exploring the principles: from the 7th International Congress of the F. M. Alexander Technique, 16–22 August 2004, Oxford, England.* STAT Books, S. pp. 85–97.

Doherty, C., Delahunt, E., Caulfield, B., Hertel, J., Ryan, J. and Bleakley, C. (2013). The Incidence and Prevalence of Ankle Sprain Injury: A Systematic Review and Meta-Analysis of Prospective Epidemiological Studies. *Sports Medicine,* 44(1), pp. 123–40. Available at: https://doi org/10.1007/s40279-013-0102-5 [Accessed 30 Mar, 2020].

Esquirol Y. (2018) Wrinkles and risk of death in a middle-aged working population. *Archives of Cardiovascular Diseases Supplements* 10(1), pp. 125–126. Available at: https://doi.org/10.1016/j.acvdsp.2017.11.163 [Accessed 30 Mar, 2020].

Harrer, G. (2017). The Fascial Distortion Model Originated by Stephen P. Typaldos. In: Liem, T., Tozzi, P. and Chila, A., eds. *Fascia in the Osteopathic Field.* Edinburgh: Handspring. Ch 35.

Jensen, M., Brant-Zawadzki, M., Obuchowski, N., Modic, M., Malkasian, D. and Ross, J. (1994). Magnetic Resonance Imaging of the Lumbar Spine in People without Back Pain. *New England Journal of Medicine,* 331(2), pp. 69–73. Available at: https://doi.org/10.1056/NEJM199407143310201 [Accessed 30 Mar, 2020].

Kasten, M. (2010). Which Way Is Up When You Are Upside Down? American Fascial Distortion Model Association. Available at: https://afdma.com/product/which-way-is-up-when-you-are-upside-down-2/ [Accessed 30 Mar, 2020].

Levenson, R. (2015). *Pigeons (Columba livia) as Trainable Observers of Pathology and Radiology Breast Cancer Images.* [e-journal] PLoS One, 10(11). Available at: https://doi.org/10.1371/journal.pone.0141357 [Accessed 30 Mar, 2020].

Liem, T., Tozzi, P. and Chila, A. (2017). *Fascia in the Osteopathic Field.* Edinburgh: Handspring.

Maher, C., Underwood, M. and Buchbinder, R. (2017). Non-specific low back pain. *The Lancet,*

389(10070), pp. 736–747. Available at: https://doi.org/10.1016/S0140-6736(16)30970-9 [Accessed 30 Mar, 2020]. Epub 2016 Oct 11.

Nagel, M. (2015). *The Fascial Distortion Model As developed by Stephen Typaldos D.O.* 1st ed. Edina, MN: Beaver's Pond Press.

Pentzer, Mitchell R. Verification of proper Greek and Latin terms. (Personal communication. 14 June, 2019)

Plint, A.C., Bulloch, B., Osmond M.H., Stiell, I., Dunlap, H., Reed, M., Tenenbein, M., and Klassen, T.P. (1999). Validation of the Ottawa Ankle Rules in children with ankle injuries. *Acad Emerg Med.* Oct; 6(10), pp. 1005–9. Available at: https://doi.org/10.1111/j.1553-2712.1999.tb01183.x [Accessed 30 Mar, 2020].

Stiell, I. The Ottawa Ankle Rules. *The Ottawa Rules.* Available at: http://www.theottawarules.ca/ankle_rules [Accessed 30 Mar, 2020].

Typaldos, S. (1994). Introducing the Fascial Distortion Model. *AAO Journal*, [online] (Spring), pp. 14–18,30–36. Available at: https://afdma.com/articles/introducing-fascial-distortion-model/ [Accessed 30 Mar, 2020].

Typaldos, S. (1994). Triggerband Technique. *AAO Journal*, [online] (Winter), pp. 15–18, 28–33. Available at: https://afdma.com/articles/triggerband-technique/ [Accessed 30 Mar, 2020].

Typaldos, S. (1995). Continuum Technique. *AAO Journal*, [online] (Summer), pp. 15–19. Available at: https://afdma.com/articles/continuum-technique/ [Accessed 30 Mar, 2020].

Typaldos, S. (2002). *Fascial Distortion Model: Clinical and Theoretical Application of the Fascial Distortion Model Within the Practice of Medicine and Surgery.* 4th ed. Orthopathic Global Health Publications.

Typaldos, S. (2017). *Fascial Distortion Model: The clinical and theoretical application of the fascial distortion model within the practice of medicine and surgery.* 25th Anniversary ed. Berrien Springs, MI: Typaldos Publishing Co.

van den Berg, F. (2017). Histology of Fascia. In: Liem, T., Tozzi, P. and Chila, A., eds. *Fascia in the Osteopathic Field.* Edinburgh: Handspring. Ch 5.

INDEX